PRAISE FO

Healing with Nature

"More keen-eyed companion than therapist, Susan Scott nudges us to look for lessons in healing that lie beyond the manicured space of therapeutic practice. With her camera and stories, she invites us to see the young maple springing from the burl, a wound on an ancient tree. Along the way, she invites us to heal that which can be healed, and perhaps more important, to carry forth with exuberant new life that which we must take on."
—James S. Korcuska, Ph.D., NCC, Resource Review Editor for Counseling Today

"How to describe this extraordinary book! Susan Scott's stunning photographs, her lovingly attentive verbal descriptions of woods like those my dogs and I walk in each morning has enabled me to notice the amazing stories embedded in the beautiful and miraculous pattern of growth of this cedar or that fir as it has responded to the particular challenges of its immediate setting and life history. She helps us see how our lives—her own, those of her patients and friends, mine—are informed by the same natural patterns, exhibit the same fierce resilience, the same quiet coming to terms."
—Christine Downing, Ph.D., author of The Goddess

"Susan Scott's Healing with Nature is a lyrical, literary journey through nature and through Jungian concepts of healing. A delightful amalgam of science, natural science, and beautiful description, Healing with Nature is about the difficult craft of being human. All those who love nature or are concerned with personal growth will find this irresistible. This is psychology in its finest form—storytelling."
—Susan Zwinger, Ph.D., author of Still Wild, Always Wild

ς

Healing
with
Nature

Susan S. Scott

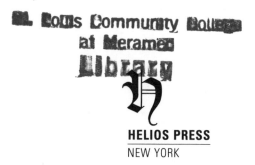

HELIOS PRESS
NEW YORK

AUTHOR'S NOTE: The stories in this book are true, and
I have been given permission to share them, but to honor
the confidentiality of clients, I have changed names and
other identifying characteristics.

For more information about the author, go to
www.susansscott.com

07   06   05   04   03
5   4   3   2   1

Published by Helios Press
An imprint of Allworth Communications, Inc.
10 East 23rd Street, New York, NY 10010

Cover and book design by Derek Bacchus

ISBN: 1-58115-303-1

Library of Congress Cataloging-in-Publication Data

Scott, Susan S.
   Healing with nature / Susan S. Scott.
        p. cm.
Includes index.
   ISBN 1-58115-303-1 (pbk.)
   1. Walking—Therapeutic use. 2. Nature, Healing power of.
   3. Psychotherapy. 4. Trees.   I. Title.
   RM727.W34S36 2003
   615.5—dc21

2003011601
Printed in Canada

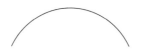

FOR RUSS

With love and gratitude

"HERE WE MUST FOLLOW NATURE
AS A GUIDE,
AND WHAT THE DOCTOR THEN DOES IS LESS
A QUESTION OF TREATMENT
THAN OF
DEVELOPING THE CREATIVE POSSIBILITIES LATENT
IN THE PATIENT HIMSELF."

C.G. JUNG,
Collected Works, Volume 16,
PARAGRAPH 82

Table of Contents

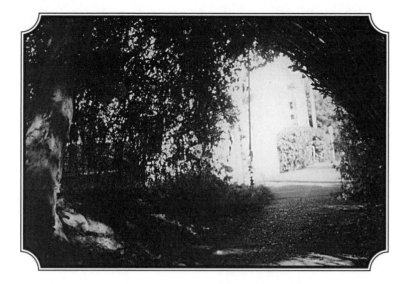

Acknowledgments

*O*ver the ten years of this book's evolution from seedling to tree, I am thankful for Russ Lockhart, artist of the soul, who walked beside me from the beginning; the Snodgrass/Mohrs for their love and belief in me, nature, and the arts; Molly and Marco for their guiding lights; Anne de Vore, Julie Gersten, Gary Hanson, Ilana Smith, Stuart Weinstein for their healing hands and hearts; Leslie Cotter and Charlotte for always being willing to play in the wild beauty of nature with me; Georgeann Johnson for the sistering spark of collaboration; Gretchen Lawlor for the jouissance of sharing *notitia* and original mind; Ned Leavitt for believing in my vision enough to help shape it into book form and represent me to publishers; Wyn Schoch, Susan Zwinger, Chris Downing, and Linda Leonard, for their passionate words and enduring support; Heather Ogilvy for sharing the wisdom of healing with her land; for the perfect timing of Ann Medlock's brilliance and book-sharing; for the soul support and humor of 5th Street Consult Group.

Julie Snyder and Sheryl Cardoza for their timely gifts of synchronicity; Meg Armstrong and Greg Lozier, for being my East Coast family and home away from home; Jim Abernathy for walking and talking with me from all over the world; the Gorman/Gilligans for sharing roots and wings; Nancy Nordhoff, staff, and fellow writers at Hedgebrook for writing time in the healing forest; Sandy Marcus for reminding me to speak for the trees; for all in my Jungian Analytic Community, particularly my mentors, Clare Buckland and Ladson Hinton; for reading the early drafts with such tender wisdom: Maddie Blais, Karin Carrington, Sharon Driscoll, Cordy Fergus, Delia Gerhard, Pui Harvey, Shira Mayer, Dick Mottern, Ann Nihlen, Jane Power, Nina Redman, Erica Richter, Lynae Slindon.

I appreciate the generosity of Jim and Molly Brown, Annapoornae Colangelo, Paul and Pat Marano, Jerry Wennstrom, Marilyn Strong, and Angie Waugur for sharing their stories; the care-filled editing of my later drafts by A.T. Birmingham-Young, Barb Connor, Jo Rothenberg, and Connie Woolf; the swift and certain legal counsel of Trudy Gasteazoros; Deb Valis and Steve Shapiro, Teri Noel, Michael and Luisa Mooney, Sharon Spencer and Marianne Mansfield for helping create public space for the tree photos; the warm-hearted tech-support of Boomerang Printing, Mary Farmer, Robert Gilman, Susan Herzerg, Kevin Upton; for seeing and loving the trees with me: Ardai Baharmast, Christina Baldwin, Kathie Lehner, Ann Linnea, Erica Moseley, Kate Nelson, Mary Rose Nuse, CJ Peterson, Phil Pearl, Mary Ellen Stone, Liza von Rosenstiel.

I am ever grateful for Tad Crawford from Allworth Press for finding my book, like a tree in the forest, and publishing it so that many others will have the chance to heal with nature; for the staff of Helios Press for being a joy to work with: Liz Van Hoose for tending the first stage of editing with gentle heart and sharp mind; Jessica Rozler for brilliant copyediting; Derek Bacchus for his artistic insight and beautiful articulation; Birte Pampel for her warm enthusiasm for introducing my book to the world.

I thank all the clients I have had the privilege to work with over the years, for they have contributed their alchemy to creating the gold that shines through all the pages of this book.

INTRODUCTION

Seeing with New Eyes

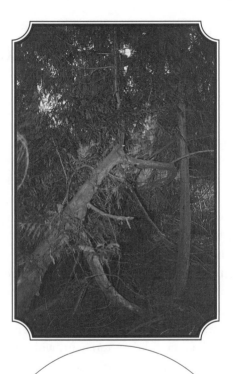

Living Castle of Trees

on hilltop overlooking meadow in

Langley, Washington.

Several species of trees cluster together, forming shelter for wildlife.

Some branches swirl or swoop to the ground,

root, then rise into trunks that

in turn branch to form protective walls.

Introduction

My pilgrimage into nature began in 1991, when a back injury forced me up and out of my chair as a writer and psychotherapist. I could not sit down without causing damage to my spinal nerves, so I either had to do walking therapy sessions with my clients or take a sabbatical from my work altogether. At the time of choosing to walk, I had no idea that my entire life would be completely and permanently changed by stepping outside my office door. Spiritual callings I knew about had to do with a gentle, but insistent, knock on the door. Mine felt like being knocked to the floor, then kicked out the door.

The first few years of healing and discovery were mostly filled with pain, fear, and disheartenment, with only glimpses of insight and new possibilities. Very gradually, over the next ten years, those brief views expanded into more enduring perspectives that changed my vision and life direction very much like trees were changed by the turning of light. This book is not only about the transformation of my work with clients and my vision as a psychotherapist; it is about how nature, trees in particular, teach us to recognize and accept the gift of healing already present in our lives. I include stories from my life, my clients', colleagues', friends', and family's lives. The chapters coincide with my discovery process as it unfolded over the decade of my pilgrimage, beginning with walking with my clients, learning about the medical world and healing back injuries, and learning how to recognize nature's healing gifts.

Seeing with New Eyes

I have written *Healing with Nature* to give everyone an opportunity to share in this new vision and the exhilaration of personal discovery. I try not to draw conclusions or preconceive for the reader, so that each person is able to do what I did: share the joy of learning from the creative process as it unfolds into the unknown. Photographs of particular trees that reveal unique shapes of growth and healing precede each chapter. The stories that follow are intended to show how people, when seen through nature's lens, heal and find their own innate genius in ways that are similar to the trees'. I invite anyone who is interested in seeing life and healing with new eyes to begin with a simple walk in the woods.

Meandering through a meadow on rural Whidbey Island one day, I noticed a cluster of trees perched like a castle on the top of a hill. Their branches appeared to be woven together, providing what looked to be a natural shelter for wildlife. I traipsed ahead, eager to see what might be inside. The tall grasses I walked through, rich with nettles and berries, revealed the imprints where deer had spent the previous night. Perhaps they were inside the cluster of trees, but I could find no easy access through a barricade of thorny blackberry vines, salmon berry bushes, and stinging nettles. I walked the perimeter until I was almost full circle, finally locating an opening under the blackberry vines where I could crawl through.

On my hands and knees I suddenly laughed out loud, recalling the *Pilgrim Astronomer*, a famous sixteenth-century woodcut of a man on his hands and knees peeking under the edge of a rainbow. Half his body was in the realm of everyday life with the village, trees, and meadows behind him; the other half reached toward the heavens. Though we were both searching other realms on our hands and knees, there was a significant difference between us. I was reaching as deeply as I could into the present moment of everyday life, into the real, not the celestial, world, looking for the healing gifts offered by nature.

Illuminated before me was an abundance of miracles of the life force made manifest in the life stories of trees. On my left,

3

running along the ground for about fifteen feet, was a cedar tree, but it had not fallen. It simply had not yet risen. I crawled all the way inside to stand up and have a look around. The cedar had to grow sideways, rather than upward, to find light, because the faster-growing alders nearby had blocked its overhead sunlight.

Clearing away the fallen branches and pine needles covering it, I noticed wavelike patterns every two or three feet along the trunk where it had attempted to rise but still couldn't find enough light. Tucking itself back to the ground, the cedar continued to stretch horizontally to the outer edges of the live canopy. Finally reaching light, it turned upward to become a standing cedar, about fifteen feet high. Altogether, it looked to be thirty feet long, half on the ground, half in the sky, creating one of the lush outer walls of the living castle.

Hardly any sunshine penetrated the overhead shelter of leaves, making it quite dark and cozy, and private enough to provide a good hideaway for wildlife. I could see why the deer would live nearby for the best of both worlds created by sun and shade. I sat down next to the long-running cedar and considered how elemental and essential these ingredients were for the living sculptures I had come to recognize. I had been thinking of light as the primary guiding force in the lives of trees, but I recognized with the long-running cedar that shade was equally vital in the sculpting process, as was true in our lives as well. When, where, and how we turned during our darkest and most challenging times truly did shape who we became as human beings. It was easy enough to grow in full light to become whatever was in our destiny, but the mix between light and dark made possible a far more creative expression of life.

Across from me was another artistic dance between sun and shade. A leaning cedar had thrust one of its branches toward the ground like a crutch to hold itself up, but the branch didn't just stop there. After dropping six feet to touch the earth and send roots into the soil, it then curved back up to form itself into a thirty-foot-tall tree. And higher up the leaning trunk, another branch, sensing this tree in its path, had radically changed its own course by curving in midair like a dancer making a pirouette on pointe. Moving laterally until it could find its own light ten feet beyond, this curving branch finally turned upward to make a tree as well. The cedar, by making several extraordinary swirls of life, had created the weaving that completed the far wall.

My view from inside the living castle proved to be magical no matter which way I turned. Like Alice in Wonderland I reveled in this wondrous world, but unlike Alice I did not have to leave my world to find it, nor did I have to swallow any mind-altering substances to see into these realms. The trees themselves had always been just as they were. It was my self and my vision that had been cracked open to see more clearly into the present-day, normal reality of time and space. A friend of mine called this way of seeing *aboriginal*, meaning that which was most original, and, most essentially for me, that which revealed meaning about the life force. This was sacred, worth bowing to like a spiritual pilgrim for a good, long look into the heart of healing.

But, as I mentioned earlier, a dark shading of despair had preceded this pilgrimage, when, on April 4, 1991, a herniated disc in my lower spine broke me open to a kind of anguish I had not yet known before in my forty-three years of living. The emergency room therapists prescribed steroids and painkillers that did not even touch the pain but made me feel very sick to my stomach. After two weeks of steadily declining, I realized that whatever had happened to me was not going to heal easily or fast—maybe not at all. Walking proved to be the only activity that did not cause me more agony. Sitting was unbearable for more than a few minutes at a time, lying down a torture because I was unable to rise or turn over without searing pain, and standing caused my back muscles to splint, so I could not bend in any direction. At first, I did not know how to begin healing when everything that happened seemed to cause further injury. I would soon discover that I would have to look beyond most of my preconceived ideas about the healing process, both physically and psychologically. I would have to learn how to see again as a beginner.

About a month after my back injury, I was limping ever so slowly and tenderly in the woods near my home in Seattle when I felt a surging sensation inside that threatened to pitch me forward into a faint, a vomit, or a sobbing heap of anguish. I could not tell which was about to happen, so I leaned up next to a tall, sturdy cedar tree and tried to breathe steadily. My stomach, scorched by the medications meant for the inflammation of my spinal nerves, was about to turn itself inside out. I was afraid to vomit, already anticipating the convulsive ripples of pain in my back. Breathing shallow and fast, almost panting, I leaned my spine up against the tree, felt its supporting spine, and in that moment the surging sensation turned into sobs. My tears felt hot, and they hurt, squeezing out of me like a washcloth being wrung dry. Everything hurt. I heard myself whisper a quivering wail to no one in particular, *Please help me.*

What followed my request—or prayer, as I eventually came to recognize that moment—was an image of tree rings and spinal discs. They appeared in my imagination spontaneously as I leaned against the tree, weeping. Tree rings and spinal discs. Concentric circles. I knew that tree rings could be counted, that they represented the seasons of a tree. One could count the number of years a tree had lived by its rings. By measuring how thick or thin those concentric rings were, one could also see how the tree had lived through years of abundance and drought. I did not yet know much about spinal discs, but I imagined that they too might have concentric circles in them. I knew they were made to flex like springs, so that the vertebrae in the spine did not rub against each other bone on bone. I knew that one of my discs was now flattened like a tire. This would be considered a drought year if it were a tree ring. My concentric line would be thin, but I hoped there would be more seasons ahead, as there were for the tree supporting my aching back. Walking slowly back home, I wondered what would happen to me.

Only in retrospect did I understand that I had surrendered my powers of healing to some other force beyond myself in that moment of excruciating pain and despair. My request had come out as a wail, unbidden. A plea for help in the midst of my anguish. I was a healer, but I needed some help beyond what I was already doing for myself, which was quite a lot at that time in my life. I had a support team of spine specialists, physical therapists, psychoanalysts, a marriage and family, friends, work I loved, and time for creative writing. In fact, there was nothing missing from my team that I knew of. Who or what did I mean by this quaking-to-the-roots cry for help? I did not know that whispering, *Please help me*, was the beginning of a pilgrimage that I would be walking for over a decade. I only knew that I needed a kind of healing I did not yet have, that my practice as a healer called for something more than I was doing.

I responded to this call by stumbling in bewilderment from my office into nature to walk side-by-side with my clients, relying on two compass points that already guided my life through unknown territory: to look carefully at what was being revealed, and above all else do no harm, the latter being primary to my profession's Hippocratic oath. After fifteen years of practice as a psychotherapist, I was prepared for *sitting with* whatever happened during sessions, but not for walking with my clients. I had to learn how to look closely at what was so, question my preconceived assumptions, then welcome the new life that followed as it did in nature.

During this time of changing vision, I came to recognize that the very practice of psychotherapy in its traditional form could be dangerous to one's health, that the devotion to maintaining certain known and accepted assumptions actually prevented some from healing. This was true for both psychotherapist and client. Besides my own struggle for health and healing, I had been a sad and helpless witness to debilitating illnesses, auto-immune disorders, and midlife deaths of too many beloved colleagues and mentors in the field of psychology. I knew these diseases to be rampant in our time and likely to have resulted at least partially from the accumulation of environmental toxins— but they happened at an alarming rate to practitioners of my profession. Something more was called for, beyond what those of us in the healing arts had learned and were practicing as wounded healers. Before I share what reaches beyond, I will first describe the essence of the wounded healer tradition and how it evolved from mythology.

The myth of the wounded healer, whose beginnings can be traced back to the ancient Greeks, provide the prototype on which most modern healing therapies are based. This prototype—symbolized by the centaur, Chiron—embodied the conflict and potential unity between the instinctual and civilized natures of human beings. Centaurs, with their powerful horse bodies and human torsos, hunted by chasing down their prey and wrestling them to the ground. They were also capable of gathering medicinal plants for healing; thus, they were known as the inventors of hunting and medicine. Such potential for both wounding and healing suggested an ethical dilemma, which was mediated by Chiron, the most celebrated of centaurs.

Originally a god, Chiron had been wounded twice before he became a centaur: first, by his mother's abandonment of him as an infant, and second, by a poisonous arrow that Hercules had intended for another. As a god his suffering would have been eternal. He made the difficult choice of becoming a mortal by trading places with Prometheus, which meant that he would experience both the pleasures and the limitations of mortality: he would have to die eventually and pass on his gifts to the next generation of mortals.

Knowing this, he lived a meaningful life by teaching what he discovered about healing, music, the arts, medicine, and ethics. He fostered many Greek heroes, including Asclepius, who became the god of healing. Chiron, as a master of the centaurs, modeled how to live in harmony with the paradox of two opposing forces at once without splitting and fighting, as was the custom of mortals and gods alike. By embodying both the wound and its healing, he became known as a wounded healer who inspired healing in others. With Chiron, the Greeks felt that gods should not be chastised for a wound or illness, because it was often through such a dilemma that one could find a deeper connection to the meaning of life, or to the divine.

Hippocrates followed Chiron's teachings with the tenet, *Physician, heal thyself*, which meant that every physician must learn to heal herself before she could heal another. Though this is no longer common practice in modern medicine, the wounded healer motif has been, without a doubt, the foundation upon which the healing arts were built. Fortunately, many of the psychoanalytic practices have continued to honor this ancient teaching, requiring trainees to go through many years of in-depth analysis and self-healing before they may work with others. This premise has been at the root of my life's work and had been effective for my clients and for me up to the time of my back injury and the beginning of my healing.

9

During the last decade of my pilgrimage into nature, I have learned how to see beyond the tradition of wounded healer into the heart of healing. I have witnessed the creative manifestations of a life force within myself, my clients and colleagues, friends, and family, no matter what stage of development we are in, no matter what kind of crisis or circumstance we face, no matter if we are thriving, just surviving, healing, even dying. Our most unique gifts can be revealed in response to situations in life that are impossible to reconcile in any ordinary or preconceived way. Something original will be required of us to grow beyond, around, or through certain situations that have befallen us, much like trees in the forest have learned to do.

At times we may struggle with an overabundance of dark, difficult periods and wonder if we will ever make it through to meaningful lives. We find that cycles of light and dark times may become a comfortable and ordinary rhythm of living. A relief. Occasionally, a great concentration of light accelerates growth so fast that we need rest, are overwhelmed, look for shade to slow down productivity a bit. No matter where we find ourselves in this dance, the creativity of our life force can be found dwelling within the heart of healing.

CHAPTER ONE
Walking Therapy

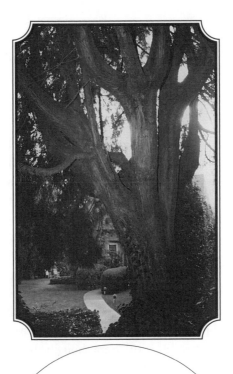

Cedar in the City,

abundant with eight separate trunks stemming

from one cedar.

Stands at the entrance of my psychotherapy building, which houses

eight offices in Seattle, Washington.

Chapter One

Sara, a forty-five-year-old single woman who had struggled with depression for most of her life, was mute and miserable in my office one day. Finding no words to express herself, she spent the first fifteen minutes crying. Then she wanted to go walking for the rest of the hour. Though I practiced walking therapy sessions almost exclusively during the first few months following my back injury, I hesitated to leave the office when clients were as vulnerable as Sara was that day. I worried about not being able to assure her privacy. My office, located in a residential section of houseboats along the shores of Lake Union in Seattle, was usually a quiet and peaceful place, but interruption from the outside world was always possible. Still, Sara thought that walking might be more helpful than just sitting in her misery. So we decided to give it a try. At least being in motion side by side offered a possibility for something different to happen. Neither of us knew what that might be, but we both felt hopeful.

When we came upon a small park along the lake shore, Sara stopped and stared at the water. Her dark, shoulder-length hair covered her face so I could not see her expression, but her attention had shifted dramatically from inside to something outside. Following her gaze, I could see ducks and seagulls on the water swimming in front of us, chattering and screeching for breadcrumbs. A mother and toddler tossed pieces from their picnic lunch, causing a flurry of wings and swirling of water as the birds scrambled for food. But Sara was not seeing any of this.

Suddenly, she whispered, her voice shimmering with awe, "That's exactly how I feel."

"How?" I said, trying to see what she meant.

Brushing the hair from her face, she said, "Look, Susan, the Canada goose is washing himself."

Beyond the food scramble, further out in the lake, I could finally see what riveted her attention. Sitting on the water, graceful as a dark swan, a very large Canada goose dipped his head underwater, then up, under and up, then a flapping of wings, and again he dipped, under and up. Looking closely now, we could both see that his movements were desperate and compulsive. He stretched up high on the water, shook himself violently, and dipped under again and again, trying in vain to wash himself clean.

Very quietly, Sara said, "He has oil on his feathers. He doesn't know how to get it off." 13

Standing helplessly by, we watched his plight, knowing he must have landed in an oil slick left by a careless boater. In that moment Sara cried.

Then she said, "That's how my depression feels. No matter what I do, it never comes off."

Acknowledging her discovery with a nod, I recognized the poignancy of her description of depression, but I also heard something different in her voice as we watched the Canada goose continue to struggle with oil on his feathers. I heard tenderness and concern, not only for the vulnerability of an animal, but also for herself. This was the first time in the two years we had worked together that she spoke of herself with love and concern instead of shame and criticism.

She turned to look at me with clear eyes, the cloudy confusion dissipated. "But I keep trying and trying just like he does. Makes me feel so sad."

My worst fear had just occurred. Our session had been interrupted, but the interruption had proven to be a gift that we might not have experienced together in any other way. Had we stayed in our chairs locked safely away from the world, Sara probably would not have found words to express her truth. The plight of a Canada goose evoked compassion, a welcome intrusion into Sara's therapy.

When our session ended, I kept my promise to note several observations. Walking side by side did make a difference in how we communicated. Sara was more spontaneous and self-expressive, less guarded, and so was I. Stepping out of our seats, which had kept us looking only at one another, our actual visual field opened up to a broader perspective. Our roles changed as well. No longer was I sitting on a throne of authority; rather, I was walking along the path with her much like a scout in the wilderness. Two with authority were learning together, though I was the more experienced guide into the unknown. By witnessing Sara's discovery in nature, I could affirm the beginning stages of a loving connection to herself, a major step in moving through her depression.

Though at first I thought Sara had projected herself onto an animal, I realized instead that she had felt deeply related to it. This is different from placing what is unconscious or unarticulated in oneself onto another in order to see it more clearly. Sara's feelings moved compassionately back and forth between her and the distressed animal. By connecting in this way to nature, she also connected to herself. Sara and the Canada goose shared a live moment in the present, though neither was in a reciprocal relationship with the other. The closest I could come to naming such a phenomenon was to call it synchronistic, because it happened at the same time without a causal connection. This was new, something beyond the familiar process in psychotherapy of working with projections. I paid close attention to what might follow.

From that moment on, Sara wanted to do walking therapy whenever the weather permitted. Most of our sessions during the following year were outdoors and involved several spontaneous encounters with the natural world, each of which eased and opened Sara's flow of self-expression. One day, at the beginning of a session, she handed me a box, beaming with confidence and joy. Opening the lid, I felt the excitement and mystery of this important moment we shared, but I could not identify the treasure wrapped carefully in cotton.

Sara laughed, "That's because you aren't around elementary schools much. It's a chrysalis. There's a monarch butterfly in there."

I was holding a precious jewel in my palm as Sara described how to place it in the sun near a window so it could fly away after the metamorphosis was complete. She explained that the cocoon provided all the nourishment necessary, and that all it needed was warmth and safety in which to grow and become its new self.

Walking and talking side by side, and encounters with nature, both contributed to Sara's growing sense of herself beyond the confines of depression. She not only became more confident and expressive during our therapy sessions; she also began to recognize, then follow, her spontaneous, creative urges to paint. One day, she came into my office and announced that we were going to spend the hour inside because she had a surprise to share. She sat down, placed a large mailing tube on her lap, then said she had painted a picture of a keening raven we had come upon during our last walking session.

I could still remember that raven because we had barely been able to hear one another over its harsh and unrelenting, but painfully urgent, *cawwww, cawwww*. We had walked over to where it perched on a telephone wire, beak open, facing the ground, throat feathers ruffling with each call. As we drew close, the raven did not fly away, did not even seem to notice our approach, but continued to *cawww* without pause at something on the ground. When we came upon a pile of black feathers strewn in the grass, we could recognize the focus of his distress and finally share the moment, rather than be distracted by it. A dead raven lay on the ground directly under the telephone wire.

We stood silently together for a long time, stunned and moved, thankful for the opportunity to bear witness to this moment in nature. Returning to the office, we continued to hear the keening, but it was no longer harsh or distracting, for we recognized it as a naturally passionate cry for the loss of life.

Sara spoke respectfully of the raven as she unrolled not one, but four paintings. We placed them side by side, covering the entire floor space between our chairs. There perched the raven on his telephone wire, but she had portrayed him watching another raven fly away into the sky. The direct simplicity of these images brought alive and amplified the natural grief, longing, and acceptance of good-bye.

The next painting revealed a young woman in profile drumming, the light of sunrise spilling over her shoulder. Sara had painted with oils, using teal-blue hues on violet-blue paper, creating an intense luminosity. Her third painting made us laugh, for there was a bear cub straddling a branch but staying as close as she could to the security of the tree trunk. Sky and leaves framed this composition in nature of a tender relationship between strength and vulnerability. Sara's fourth painting portrayed a high-corner angle of an adobe home with a clear southwestern sky, backlighting and contrasting with the soft edges of brown adobe. A ladder connected one roof to another, giving a feeling of motion to an otherwise static, esthetically beautiful scene.

Sara said, "I was surprised at how fast I could paint these and how happy I was. For most of the time I painted. Even now, looking at them, I feel in-love feelings."

We had walked from the office through a threshold into the mystery and gift of healing with nature. For this I felt thankful. I understood those in-love feelings that involved not another person but a mysterious, creative phenomenon. It had to do with being related to the natural cycles of life, death, then new life. I, too, experienced that surge of in-love feelings when standing in front of trees that inspired new life for me, and was often moved to make a photograph of them just as Sara was moved so passionately to represent her healing images through her paintings.

As a psychotherapist, part of being in relation to the natural cycles of life, death, and regeneration meant being present for each stage of each client's transformational process. Not everyone wanted to do walking therapy in spite of the fact that it was better for me than sitting. This meant I had to deal very directly with a phenomenon called "countertransference," which has to do with the unresolved issues a therapist might project onto her client. Usually, issues of transference work the other way around—from client to therapist. We are trained to pay attention to both possibilities and ask for consultation from other psychotherapists when the need arises.

I asked for a consultation right after I'd received my diagnosis of the herniated disk. The psychologist I consulted pointed out that my wound and how I dealt with it could be seen as a gift, not a burden, to clients, and that it is not often a client is given the opportunity to witness firsthand how the therapist relates to her own healing. He believed my clients might learn more about healing from this window of our experience together, even benefit greatly from it, depending on how I worked with my own psychology. Another way to put this was: I had a chance to practice what I preached about healing. The key was to listen closely to myself and my clients, and be willing to step into uncharted territory for the answers.

Though walking with my clients eventually brought us closer to the mystery and gift of healing, at first we were all apprehensive about leaving the office. We simply had to learn together, feeling our way in the dark, sometimes not finding light for a long time. For the first few months following my back injury, my life and work seemed to be a dangerous and exhilarating dance between dark and light. I made extraordinary discoveries in the process, which made me grateful, yet the pain in my back not only persisted, it grew worse. My wound would not allow me to sit for more than fifteen minutes at a time without causing damage to the spinal nerves controlling movement of my legs.

I let each of my clients choose whether or not he or she wanted to do walking therapy with me, but when they chose to stay in the office, I had to worry about their witnessing my pain, about the impact of pain on my concentration, about their feelings of doing therapy with a clearly wounded therapist. Should I take a sabbatical from working altogether? How would such a sudden disruption affect my clients? How could I do it financially? Should I change careers? Was this what my healing was going to require of me? Until I could answer such questions, I had clients scheduled to see me, and I simply had to do the best I could with each and every person. From hour to hour, I did not know whether I would be walking or whether I would have to squirm and alternate positions in the office, all the while trying to focus on our conversation, not on my own pain.

I learned that I could squat longer than I could stand or be on the kneeling chair. Standing proved to be only slightly less painful than sitting and was the most exhausting of all. Though squatting gave my back the most relief, my knees couldn't tolerate such a stance for more that fifteen to twenty minutes at a time. Exhaustion became a most serious consideration for managing chronic pain. After several office sessions in a row, I would lie down on the floor during my break, with a pillow under my knees, and either fall asleep or cry. Often both my body and my feelings felt profoundly hurt.

With some clients in my therapy practice, the decision not to walk was an important part of developing a therapeutic relationship. It was an essential stage of development for one of my clients, who had been sexually abused by her previous therapist. She needed safe containment and consistency more than she needed exploration via walking therapy. I had been carefully building such a trusting environment with her over the months preceding my injury and did not want to introduce anything that might threaten the boundaries she was rebuilding.

Unfortunately, she had been one of the many clients whose session I had to cancel the first week of my injury.

The best we could do was talk about it honestly when she struggled with fears of abandonment and her ambivalence toward psychotherapy. Neither of us knew for sure whether it would work, but we were willing to try. Truthfulness had a sacred place in her therapy this time, as did working with a wounded healer who was trying desperately to heal herself. The success of my work with her over time had as its foundation the capacity to live with opposing forces at once. She discovered that she was able to safely experience being both compassionate and frightened, protective of herself and concerned for me in the office.

Depending on what each client needed to do within the therapeutic alliance we had created together, there was a wide range of responses that seemed to match the spring weather: stormy, then clear, and stormy once again. Sometimes we walked, sometimes we did not. Until each client came to his or her session and we discussed whether or not we would be doing walking therapy that day, I did not know whether we would be outside or inside for therapy.

Each client was different. A middle-aged man who seemed constricted when in his chair was looser and quite a bit more relaxed while walking and talking. He would put on his hat before we walked out the door, reminding me of the carefree image of the Fool in the Tarot Deck, open and happy to be having an adventure into the unknown with me by his side. Another client, who was bulimic, returned from a half-hour walk with me to say how happy she felt not to have thought about her body image the whole time we were talking. Usually, she was extremely self-conscious about other people's glances in public, but she sensed there had been a *bubble of safety* around us as we walked down the sidewalk together.

Still another client refused to try walking therapy. The predominant feeling during the first session we shared following my back injury was of his watchfulness and wariness of me.

I think he must have been hypersensitive to any chance of not being seen or heard because of my pain. He wasn't going to allow a minute of it, having been raised and severely neglected by an alcoholic mother. By the end of the first session, I remember feeling that I had barely passed the test of not being like his mother, who had never listened to him. Lucky for us, my capacity to hear with empathy was not compromised as I stood, squatted, and sat with him through the hour.

Yet I also remember how tense I had felt, because he had been one of the few clients who seemed furious at me for being injured. I was desperate for another consultation, but I still could not sit long enough to make the hour-long drive to see my psychologist in those early months. Fortunately, my partner was able to take time off from work and drive me to my appointment. I remember lying in the back of the car to save my sitting time for consultations, mostly worrying about my impact on clients and the wound's impact on my own psychology. I wanted to understand a nightmare: I had been stung by a scorpion. I had almost died and was feeling very sick. What would Chiron do in this situation? Though I felt inspired by the wounded healer motif, I was also just beginning to recognize how devastating my back injury was and how long it might take to heal.

CHAPTER TWO
Wounded Healer

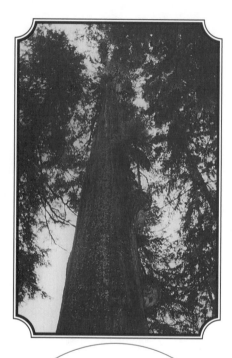

New Life *grows*

in an old-growth forest on the trail to

Heather Lake

in the North Cascade Mountains, Washington. From a burl bulging

along its trunk,

a young maple tree is thriving.

Chapter Two

What actually happened to cause my back injury? A long degenerative process suddenly became acute when the spinal disc in my lower back herniated. I sank slowly, like a tire flattening down to its rim, into agony I feared might last a lifetime. My rupture was located in the disc between lumbar vertebrae 4 and 5, which on my five-foot, eleven-inch frame was just below waist level, the pivotal center from which a forward bend was made. Unbeknownst to me, it had been degenerating over several years when, with no warning signs I could have comprehended ahead of time, it burst forth to press against the nerves in my spinal column.

The night before this happened, I had gone with my partner to see the musical *Les Miserables*. Having sat with clients all day, I had been unable to find a comfortable position in the theater seat for the four hours of the show. Though I'd enjoyed the musical, when it was finally over and I stepped out of the theater into the cool night air, letting my body stretch and move in open space, I felt as if I had just been released from prison. The next morning, I enjoyed my three-mile walk around Green Lake in Seattle, to be followed by breakfast with a friend. I had not anticipated that our conversation would lead to my crying over breakfast, heartbroken about not having been able to conceive a child. I had been sharing the parenting of my partner's children for the past ten years, but I still yearned to give birth to a child.

Only recently had I begun to realize that my biological time for a healthy pregnancy might have already passed before I was psychologically ready to let go of my dream. The conversation with my friend in the cafe that morning had touched off a reservoir of grief that surprised both of us.

When my rainstorm of tears broke open, I leaned forward and placed both elbows on the table, reaching my hands up to wipe the tears and cradle my face all at once. I sobbed softly into my hands, shaking only slightly, when I felt or heard a little pinging sensation in my lower back. Not until I leaned back against the chair, then tried to get up, did I realize that something very serious had just occurred in my body, something that would set into motion profound and bewildering life changes over the next several years. As with my spine, the structure of my whole life had begun to transform before I knew what was happening.

After our conversation, I stood up with great difficulty and drove home to prepare for my day of work. Getting in and out of the car increased the growing discomfort I felt in my lower back. This kind of pain was not new to me. Something similar had occurred three times before over the past fifteen years, but always followed strenuous exercise, careless bending, or heavy lifting. That morning I had done nothing but walk around a lake I had circumnavigated hundreds of times before, then had breakfast with a friend and shared an emotional conversation. Could this be what was meant by psychosomatic? Though my pain centered from my lumbar spine, I sensed a most significant interaction between my emotional and my physical pain.

Over the next few months I would discover, through my struggle to heal from what was finally diagnosed as a degenerative spinal condition, that herniated discs were comparable to threadbare socks. Though there might only be the tiniest little threads that were worn out or broken at the tip, eventually a toe would pop through the hole that opened up from overuse or too much pressure from inside. Such an injury within a disc was most likely to happen from the acute force of an accident or fall, or the sudden compression of lifting more than the body could tolerate. Mine had been degenerating from the chronic compression of long hours of sitting, along with the physical fact that I was a tall, slender woman. It turned out that many people with long spines, particularly athletes, often incurred lower back injuries because of the increased compression of simply bending forward.

Herniated discs could not regenerate, but they eventually would scar over to prevent further leakage. Once damaged, they could not bounce back like the springy cushion they were meant to provide for the spine. Healthy discs are like shock absorbers, protecting the vertebrae from rubbing bone to bone, or worse, crashing into one another every time we sit down. They give us a smooth ride while also preventing real structural damage that would certainly occur without them. At the time of my injury, I did not know any of this—only that the unrelenting pain in my back, like an acute toothache in the very center of me, shattered my previous vision of the healing process, made me a beginner again. I had to learn through trial and error what increased and decreased pain, what furthered my healing and what set me back, when to take medication and when to bypass it, how to trust my intuitions and when to ask for help.

25

I put together a team of medical professionals to help me learn more about the healing interaction between mind, body, and spirit. Along with a spine specialist and physical therapist, I found support in the healing arts with massage, chiropractic work, acupuncture for pain management, cranio-sacral work, and advice from a naturopath on ways to build up my health with herbs and vitamins. My life was suddenly absorbed with walking therapy sessions for my clients and for myself, paired with a seemingly endless schedule of appointments with my support team of healers. Reflecting on it now, I think I would have paced myself better had I known that my physical healing would take years, not months. When a disc blows between vertebrae, the entire back must eventually learn to adjust and compensate for the structural change that affects all parts branching from the spinal column: ligaments, nerves, arms, legs, neck, and head.

Once I understood how essential walking was to my own healing, I walked as often as I could. My friends began to invite me for strolls, rather than coming over for dinner or going out to the movies. Gratefully, within three months, I was able to take my first hike up to Heather Lake in the North Cascade Mountains. I felt happy to be moving, but not yet sturdy and confident on my feet. My friend and I moved slowly up the path that would take us to the lake. Already the trail ascended more steeply than I had anticipated. I was out of condition but pleased to discover that uphill walking did not hurt my back. I liked feeling the sweat on my skin and seeing a clear, blue sky overhead with forest all around us as we shuffled along slowly and steadfastly as inchworms. Within two hours we had climbed to the place in the trail where logging was not possible. It was like stepping into an ancient kingdom to suddenly be among the giant trees of an old-growth forest. We passed several immense old cedars whose trunks were easily ten feet or more in diameter. Their age and strength took my breath away. I *oohed* and *aahed* with my friend at every turn, until we came upon the most majestic sight of all. We stood absolutely still and stared in awe.

Towering over a hundred feet into the sky, a great cedar stood before us. A third of the way up its trunk protruded a *herniation*, or burl. From that protrusion grew another tree standing close to fifteen feet tall and as sturdy and healthy as any young tree on the ground. I stood with that wise old cedar for a long time, asking for guidance to do in my life what it had done. I, too, wanted to find a way to bring forth new life from my injury. But how? The pain seemed to be stopping me from doing things, creating endless new obstacles for me. The burl that had sprung from my spine had certainly caused me more frustration than inspiration. As a matter of fact, depression had begun to creep in around the edges of my fear and unrelenting back pain.

But the tree I stood beside infused me with hope and possibility. The cedar was a living example not only of how to grow beyond the injury, but how to support new life as well. As I continued my hike that day, I tried to imagine what kind of new life my injury could support. It seemed obvious once I opened my eyes to see what was already new and different in my life: walking with clients.

In that moment I decided to pay more attention to what actually happened during our walks rather than spend so much time worrying about whether or not we were doing the right thing. Perhaps we would discover something new together. What had been bothering me about the field of psychotherapy even before my back injury was the feeling that my work sequestered both the client and me away from life. Though I cared deeply for each of my clients, sometimes I could hardly bear to walk into my office, close the door, and sit down face-to-face for an hour-long encounter. Clearly we were closing out the world so we would not be interrupted, intending to make a safe space in which to do our work together. But I did not feel like spending such long hours just sitting in a chair talking about life. During my days off I often felt like a child on summer vacation, finally free to explore the world as it was, not as my school defined it. 27

Yet I had always considered therapy to be akin to a school or laboratory for learning how to live more fully, a place to safely develop and practice new skills. The structured sense of therapy, with its protective boundaries, underscored this idea. There were agreed-upon rules to the process, usually fifty- to sixty-minute sessions, fees, regularly scheduled hours, cancellation policies, rules of confidentiality, and consent to treatment. Based on this premise, my role as therapist had been like that of a teacher or lab scientist, and it would not be appropriate to live in a school or a lab. After all, I wanted to go home and live my own life fully with my family, and pursue my own dreams, too. I had always made a conscious division between my work and personal life, but such a division amplified the need to *get out of school* when

I was working, and the reverse when not. Even before my back injury, I had no longer wanted to go into my office and shut the classroom door on the world.

I began to wonder why I asked my clients to do therapy in my office, sequestered away from their worlds. I knew this kind of question was not likely to be well-received by a therapeutic community dedicated to and trained in the traditional practice of sitting face-to-face in an office for an hour of dialogue. Modern psychotherapy had been called the *talking cure* because of this, though there were certainly variations on this theme with hypnosis, movement therapy, and art therapy, in which sitting face-to-face in dialogue was not a primary focus. Walking therapy, on the other hand, could be practiced in nature. What was encountered would then become part of the healing process. The shape of a tree, or the weather, or the meow of a cat on the sidewalk, or the sweat on one's brow—all of these moments were part of walking therapy. Without walls, nature and the relationship between client and therapist would be what held meaning and contained the experience. I imagined myself to be more closely aligned with the sense of being a wilderness scout or guide interested in exploring the terrain, all the while honoring each client's particular and unique interest and orientation. I learned later that this was one of the steps along the way of training to be a Jungian analyst: to become a companion to the soul on its path. Walking therapy might be essential and generative for both the clients and for me, complete in itself like a poem—not a preparation for something else, but a phenomenon that brought us naturally into the world rather than sequestering us away from life. Perhaps this was the new life that wanted to be born from my back injury. The tree with another tree growing from its herniation or burl inspired me to look for new life in this way.

Such inspiration emerged from an I-thou relationship with nature, similar to what I had witnessed between my client and the Canada goose that had been desperate to wash off the oil

28

from his feathers. Sara had felt compassion for the struggle that both she and the animal were synchronistically sharing, though their actual life struggles were unique to each. And my inspiration for healing came from getting to know the life histories of each particular tree. I was not projecting my preconceived vision onto them but observing closely what they were revealing about their own lives. I appreciated the essence of tree as tree, not as symbol for something else. I was interested in the concrete details that caused its life story to take a unique shape, and I believed it had a meaningful story to share about the wisdom of the life force in all beings. I wanted to learn all that nature was willing to teach.

Nature as Mentor

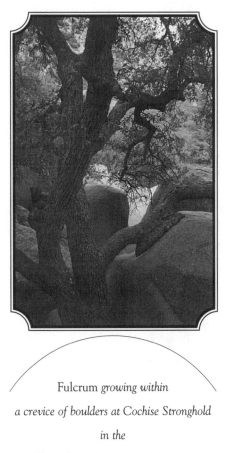

Fulcrum *growing within*
a crevice of boulders at Cochise Stronghold
in the
Chiracahua Mountains of Arizona.
This tree extends a branch laterally, using a boulder to hold its weight.

Chapter 3

Nature showed me how to reach for the light and how to make creative use of all resources available to further the life force, no matter what circumstances I found myself in, no matter how big the obstacles might have seemed at first. I closely observed the way trees incorporated into their lives whatever was in their paths, then made the best of what they found there. They became mentors, teaching by the example of their lives much like artists will do with their apprentices.

I wanted to share these gifts with my clients.

Rose, a married, thirty-four-year-old woman who had completed residential treatment for depression, told me she wanted to practice in her life what she had learned while in the hospital. Besides hoping to stay healthy and fit, Rose thought that having her body in motion during our walking therapy sessions might help her be more conscious of her body's sensations. She wanted to develop some harmony between the conflicting desires of mind, body, and soul. At first we experimented with half-hour sessions, returning to the office to discuss impressions of the experience. After several weeks of doing our walking therapy in the neighborhood around my office, she decided to commit to doing a whole year of walking sessions. We both wanted to let more of the natural world surround us than what was available in the residential neighborhood, so I considered scheduling our sessions in Carkeek Park in North Seattle. It had already become one of my weekly personal pilgrimages for healing, and I thought it might also be a good walking therapy location for clients. There were a number of interesting trees along the way which had become touchstones and resting spots for me. I decided to time myself, walking the meandering mile that traversed the hillside down to a stream emptying into Puget Sound. If it took an hour, then it might be a perfect walking therapy trail for Rose and others.

Following a path along the stream called *Salmon to Sound*, I crossed a bridge where two streams converged, coming upon a small apple orchard sloping down the hillside on my right. There were close to fifty trees in various forms of life and decay, gnarled and ancient. Leaving the trail, I walked across the orchard to see how one of the apple trees sustained its life after experiencing what could have been a mortal blow. There were pink blossoms growing from the branches on its main trunk and white blossoms coming from its secondary trunk. The splash of pastels it left against a sapphire spring sky overhead made me want to linger awhile. It looked as if the secondary trunk started growing fairly close to the base, only a foot or so up from the ground, then was cracked almost completely in half some time ago. It must have fallen to the ground and continued to grow until it stretched about six feet from the main trunk. By some miracle the broken tree trunk sent roots down into the ground, turned itself at a right angle to support its weight, and grew upright and parallel to the main tree. The secondary trunk seemed to have become a separate tree, no longer dependent on the main trunk for nurturance.

I noticed how quiet and protected I was from the sounds of the city that surrounded me on the hillside above. The steep ravine rising on both sides was covered with dense undergrowth and towering trees, filling my senses with a sound garden of bird song, wind in the trees, a rushing stream. I was about to pass the water treatment plant, which meant I was almost to the main entrance of the park. As the trail curved to the right, I crossed

33

a bridge over two more con-verging streams, which were protected with a fence and signs requesting special tend-ing of this place where the salmon spawned.

The wild ravine had given way to an open mead-ow tended by the Parks Department. I noticed that the grass was carefully groomed and there were pic-nic tables and garbage cans strategically located not too far from the parking lot. People were playing Frisbee, walking dogs, waxing their cars, bird-watching, sitting in lounge chairs reading. Some were listening to music in their cars. I continued to

34

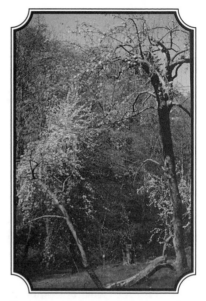

Regeneration *began life as one apple tree. One of its lower branches was broken and fell to the ground, where it rooted to create an apple tree with blossoms of a different color.*

walk beside the stream meandering along the base of a steep hill-side on my left. Through the trees I saw crisscrossing the hillside a network of trails. Stepping under a natural canopy of leaves over the path, the next five minutes of my walk were sheltered from the sun in what felt to be a mini–rain forest. The light reflected up from the wet leaves instead of from overhead. This gave a brief luminous sense of otherworldliness before I emerged into the sunlight again and the wide-open space of Puget Sound. The stream moved purposefully through a channel carved into the coarse, gray sand to finally mingle with the vast body of the sound that in turn would empty into the Pacific Ocean. The salmon needed this particular balance of salt and clear water to help them make the biological changes for their eventual survival in the ocean.

I began the ascent up a trail that led to the hilltop, where I had a better view of the islands and the Olympic Mountains in the distance. I came upon an old oak tree growing on the very edge of the bluff. Its gnarled, roughly beautiful trunk leaned at a sixty-degree angle over the escarpment. I admired its strength and age, guessing it to be several hundred years old by the width of its trunk at base. Circling around to the side facing the Sound, I discovered that most of its base was actually a hollowed-out cave. The inside was charred black, indicating a fire at some point in its life story. Perhaps lightning had struck into its foundation.

I wondered how the oak could have survived such a trauma and continued to thrive, carrying its life force over fifty feet upward into the heavens. How had it healed from such a burn? Or, had it just found a way to grow around and beyond its wound? Looking closely at what was before me, I noticed that the outer bark had grown around all the outside edges of the wound so that it appeared to be sealed, though the inside of the cave was just charred wood. The outside edges appeared to be growing downward into the roots, which were the size of elephant legs, balancing at the cliff's edge the enormous weight of this huge oak. Finally, I understood the wide girth of this tree at base as I stepped inside to consider the phenomenon of its healing. 35

With sunlight reflecting like diamonds from the water below, I reveled in the warm breeze rustling the leaves overhead, and I felt soothed by the soft repetitive sound, the expansive view with its multi-variant shades of blues, violets, and silver of the distant mountains, the clouds and sky, and the vast, live, and undulating waters of Puget Sound. I felt secure and warm with my back nestled against the tree cave.

The word *temenos*, meaning "sacred space" or "safe space for healing," was one of the primary tenets of psychotherapy. Both client and therapist needed such a space in which to do their work together. I thought of my client Rose and what she had said about our relationship being such a temenos, how safe she felt when we walked together. She also told me that her eating

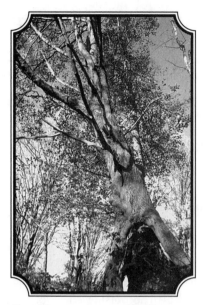

Cave Tree *growing on a bluff in Carkeek Park, Seattle, Washington, was hit by lightning years ago. This maple tree continued to grow in spite of the gaping hole left at its base.*

36

disorder had felt like a black hole that no amount of food, psychotherapy, or love could ever fill. I wondered what she would see in this magnificent oak tree rising above its dark hole, and in that moment I decided to go ahead and schedule one of our walking sessions in this park. She, too, wanted to grow into the fullness of her being, as this tree was doing, in spite of her deep wound at foundation. Over the years she had tried endless numbers of interventions and psychotherapies from a variety of theoretical orientations. I wondered if all she really needed to learn now was how to grow beyond what could not actually heal. Perhaps traditional psychotherapy itself had become just another attempt at filling the insatiable hole, only making her feel more inadequate. I had found the most healing therapy so far had been to provide the temenos, the safe and protected ground from which she could naturally grow into her own unique self, just as this tree was also doing.

What many of us psychotherapists have tended to forget at times is that a theory of healing is only a particular lens through which to see, to gather a certain kind of information that can be ordered, defined, discussed, and named, and from which a treatment plan can be decided upon. Meanwhile, the client is simply in the midst of her life's story, trying to live as best she can, just as the trees in this forest are doing.

As I contemplated these ideas, nestled comfortably inside the tree cave, I felt certain that the life story of this oak offered a gift of understanding and mentoring human healing beyond the screen of theoretical lenses. It had found a way to thrive in spite of what appeared to be a mortal wound. How? What kind of process had it gone through after the fire to preserve its life force?

Descending gradually, I followed crisscrossing trails to an old-growth stump over twenty feet high and ten feet in diameter. Thick roots descending from the top appeared to drape two tree legs down both sides of the stump. Stepping back, I noticed that those strong roots were nourishing a lone hemlock tree already standing over forty feet tall. There were many other roots weaving through and into the stump from which they nursed. But the two largest, most visible roots along the outside had transformed their cells from root to trunk cells in order to provide stability for the tree high above. They truly had become tree legs. The hemlock, in anticipating that the old-growth stump would eventually decay away from under it, naturally developed an alternate route for survival. I wondered how many years it might take for the stump to disappear completely, leaving the hemlock to stand on its own twelve-foot-long legs and appear to be like a tree walking through the forest.

The next week, when Rose and I had our first walking session in the park, she found a ponderosa pine tree I had not even noticed during my initial stroll on my own. For the first several sessions, she returned to the path that lead across the bridge and up the hill to her "mother tree," as she had named it. When standing with Rose by this mentoring tree, I felt myself listening for something to awaken in her. Rather than problem-solve the endless list of wrong things in her life, I could just begin to hear the buds of regeneration deep inside her beginning to blossom, awakening the life force that drives all of life—mine, hers, the trees. I felt a solid sense that love stood with us in the forest. Perhaps this was the essence of Mother Nature. There was a presence of something more mysterious and expansive than either of us and our therapy could do by ourselves in the office.

During one of our sessions, it started to rain lightly. We considered going back until we realized that the ponderosa pine, her "mother tree," would shelter us completely with its umbrella of branches. Rose led us to her tree, telling me that she had kept a good balance between taking care of self and *doing* too much. We stopped and listened to the rain. She said she loved the sound, that it reminded her of being a kid camping out with her father and listening to the rain on the tent together. Since the previous week, the vegetation had grown into the trail, creating an archway for us to duck under before we reached Rose's tree. Walking

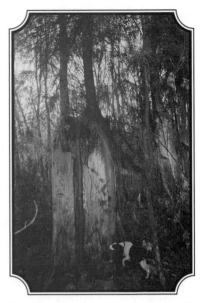

Like Trees Walking *was likely planted by a squirrel or bird who inadvertently dropped a seed at the top of an old-growth* nurse-log *in Carkeek Park, Washington. Its roots, which stand twenty feet tall, give this hemlock the appearance of a tree walking through the forest.*

through the canopy, we noticed that it was completely dry under the tree. She sighed, leaned against her touchstone, and dropped her pack to the ground. She had brought both her journal and a jug of water.

Rose said, "I imagined my tree several times this week. I moved slower. My rhythm felt more neutral. I thought of the tree and forest moving slowly, and I slowed down inside."

She talked about looking in the mirror and seeing something she appreciated about herself. For the first time, she could remember not automatically thinking how gross she looked. Instead, she noticed the color and tone of her skin and liked her healthy, ruddy complexion.

Rose asked me if I read the weekly personal ads and whether I knew what "HWP" stood for.

No, I didn't.

She said, "It stands for "height-weight-proportionate.""

Then she described other abbreviations, for words like white, male, single, female, no smoking, drugs, alcohol, and cats.

"This is how I would advertise myself," she said. "HWP— NOT ME! I'm a full bodied, full-spirited woman available!"

We laughed in celebration of her.

She added, "Look out there, Susan," indicating the woods in front of us, "Do you see even one HWP tree out there? Some are missing branches, some are leaning, twisted, nonsymmetrical, tall and thin, tall and wide, short and gnarled, every which way but HWP."

CHAPTER 4

Support for the Jouney

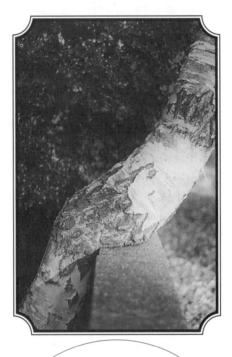

Support *made use of a low-lying wall*
that stood in the way, growing around and over it.
This birch tree
continues to thrive in the Lake City neighborhood,
north of Seattle, Washington.

Chapter 4

After two months of focused work on my own healing and doing walking therapy sessions with clients, I felt stronger and able to sit for longer than fifteen minutes at a time, but I began to notice a new and constantly burning ache in the center of my left thigh. My bone felt like it was a smoldering hot coal. I had no relief, whether I stood, sat, or lay down. Walking was the only activity that mitigated the pain at all, but by then I had trouble lifting my left foot. My leg had weakened so much that I was more worried about it than my back. When I walked with my dogs each morning, even the slightest tug on their leashes threatened to knock me off my feet. I had to concentrate on making sure my leg wouldn't buckle, which frightened the wits out of me. My physical therapist measured and tested the strength in both legs and found an inch difference in the calf and thigh muscles of my left leg as well as a 60 percent deficit in strength compared to my right leg. The muscles had atrophied. He suspected that the herniated disc was impinging on my sciatic nerve, and he suggested I call the spine specialist right away.

The most frightening moment of my entire healing process occurred in the doctor's office that day. I described the weakness in my leg. He asked me to sit up on the table and dangle my legs down, then resist his pressure as he pushed my foot down. I resisted, while he easily pushed my foot down. It no longer followed my commands. I asked to try again, thinking I had not concentrated hard enough. This time I gave it all my focus and strength, and watched my foot collapse as if it belonged to someone else. Then he tried pushing down on my big toe as I resisted. It folded over like a noodle.

He gasped, "You don't just feel weaker—you *are* weaker."

Terrified, I heard my voice shaking as I asked, "What can I do?"

I didn't want to hear that the damage might be irreversible. My tears leaked down my cheeks as I listened to him explain that the nerve damage probably came from inflammation of my sciatic nerve. He wanted to schedule an *epidural* as soon as I could do it. What was that? I felt my body quivering with this conversation. An injection of cortisone would be shot directly into my spine. "Why?" I croaked. The cortisone would reduce inflammation immediately, taking pressure off my sciatic nerve, which controlled the movement of my legs. Was there permanent damage to my nerve? Would it all come back?

Probably.

Why not definitely?

We'll just have to see. Take one step at a time.

I wished I could. What would be the next step?

A *Magnetic Resonating Image* to see exactly what the disc looked like.

Why don't we do that right now?

He explained very slowly, as if to a baby, that he treated backs, not pictures of backs. Fine, but what was wrong with seeing how it looked? It was very expensive and might not help us decide what to do next. He wanted to treat my symptoms as they expressed themselves, not whatever the picture would show on the MRI. He went on to say that some people have herniated discs but never have any symptoms. I didn't know what to say about that.

There was an immediate and undeniable truth before me now. My sciatic nerve had to stop being inflamed or I would eventually lose the use of my left leg. Hopefully, my loss could be reversed in time. We scheduled the epidural for the next afternoon at the hospital. I couldn't imagine how it might be more traumatic than the moment I watched the doctor push my foot down while I resisted. After canceling my last few clients of the day, I went to the hospital with my partner. The doctor said it was essential for someone to drive me home after the procedure, which alerted me to possibilities of this being worse than just an injection.

As we walked into the waiting room, a sobbing woman trudged out. I filled out the forms and stood by the wall, listening to my heart beating unusually fast. I wondered what could be so awful about an injection unless the doctor made some kind of terrible mistake, maybe hit her spinal cord or something. He had advised me the day before about the risks: one of which could be an allergic reaction to the dye he would inject into the spinal column, the other was the possibility of infection. He added that he had done over two thousand epidurals and had never caused either problem. I thought the odds were so small as to be unnecessary for advisement, but as I listened to the woman's sobs, I thought twice about doing it.

The strange nervy sensations in my left leg motivated me to do whatever possible to take care of the pressure on my sciatic nerve—*now!* I walked down the hallway, where I changed into a gown and waited for the doctor. I decided not to pretend bravery, and just let him know I was worried. I told him it would help me get through it if I could see exactly what he was doing. What I saw immediately were two syringes with eight- to ten-inch-long needles. I asked why they had to be so long. I had imagined he would be giving me a shot directly into the wounded disc. He showed me how the needle would enter the base of my tailbone and run along the inside of my spinal column to deliver the *medicine* six to eight inches above. He wanted to coat the sciatic nerve with cortisone all along the way to reduce the inflammation wherever it occurred.

The sensation was not so much painful as extremely odd.

Pressure is the best description, a kind of unrelenting pressure in the tailbone area, like something might explode. It was unrelenting even after the needle was withdrawn. I could understand why the other woman sobbed. She had to release the pressure somehow. I did not cry until we were home. The doctor had been very kind, patient, reassuring through the entire procedure, but intrusion into my body had somehow profoundly hurt my feelings no matter how nicely it had been done. I did not want any of this to be happening to me in the first place.

In reflection, I must have had an emotional response to cortisone. For the next ten days I was devastatingly depressed and in despair. This had also happened after the first week of my injury, when I was taking prednisone for inflammation. It was either an allergic reaction to steroids or a feeling of reinjury upon discovering the damage to my sciatic nerve—or both. I felt like I had caused harm to myself even when I tried so hard to heal. Why had I not known about the sciatic nerve problem? The doctor told me that nerves did not hurt when they were injured like muscle and other tissue, so I would not know unless I started losing strength in the muscle—as I had. This was not reassuring. He emphasized the importance of keeping down the inflammation around my disc so the sciatic nerve would not become more inflamed. This would mean no sitting at all, which was next to impossible. And so I walked.

I asked the trees to show me how to tend my left leg, which was withering like a dead branch. They might teach me to heal, I thought. They knew how to go on growing around or through or in spite of their broken branches, gashes in their trunks, severe burns, even the loss of their tops to lightning or high winds. They gave me inspiration and a sense of comfort and confidence in a healing process that was beyond my own will and effort.

One afternoon, as I strolled through the woods surrounding an abandoned army base, a group of trees caught my eye. They looked like living ladders. Boards had been nailed crossways into them to about thirty feet up each trunk. Dark sap stains dripped down from where they had bled from their wounds, but the trees had thrived beyond their nail holes. The bark of every tree had grown up and over the edges of each board so that it looked as though the trees were eating the ladders that had been built years ago by those who had inhabited the army base. What a creative solution, I thought. Rather than bleed to death, the trees had emanated enough life force to grow over their wounds, to incorporate them. Plenty of soldiers must have come to a similar solution when they had to choose whether to live with or try to remove shrapnel from their wounds. Some of the boards were almost completely absorbed by the trees, as if the ladders were being gobbled up slowly but surely over time.

Whether to intervene or incorporate is often a critical question in the healing process, whether in physical or mental health. In my case, I felt desperate not to intervene with back surgery because of the horror stories I had heard about the secondary problems that almost always resulted. Yet, as time ticked by and the strength in my left leg did not come back, I began to feel equally desperate to stop the nerve damage in any way I could. As soon as I could. Even with dreaded surgery, if necessary. But my medical doctor had recommended that we wait and see what effect the epidural of cortisone would have on the inflammation of my spinal nerves. By the end of the following week, I panicked, having sensed no difference in the strength of my leg in spite of all the walking I had done on my own and with clients. Help!

I called my doctor and was even more frightened to hear how surprised he was that the cortisone had had no effect. He wanted to know exactly what the herniated disc was doing inside my spinal column now. It was then that he scheduled an MRI, which would create a detailed photograph of organs, bones, cartilage, and discs inside the human body by blasting it within a magnetically resonating field. On the day of my MRI, I parked in front of the clinic and checked in at exactly 6:15 P.M. My hands shook as I filled out the forms and took off all of my jewelry, as the nurse requested. Since I would be in a strong magnetic force field, I had to make certain that no metal was left anywhere on my body. But my naturopathic doctor had inserted metal clips through the cartilage in my ears. How could I remove them? As I twisted and tugged at the clips, trying to imagine what held them in, I pictured ripping flesh like fish hooks, leaving me bleeding all over the front desk. Luckily, they popped out with only a minimum of trauma and no blood.

After changing into a hospital gown, I was ready to be inserted into the coffin-like contraption. The radio technician tried to prepare me for the racket of sound I would hear and the timing of it all, which would be between forty-five minutes and an hour, depending.

"Depending on what?" I asked.

Depending on what they found and whether they had to do any of it over, which depended on how still I could be. No problem there, I decided. The room was space-age, sterile, and bright. The huge machine stood in the center of the floor with a round opening two feet in diameter, where my body would be delivered into its mouth on a sliding tray. Until that very moment I had not even considered claustrophobia as a problem, probably because I had never seen such a machine before. The radiologist assured me that he would be able to talk with me through a microphone while I was in there. Yes, and I could talk to him. This meant my head would be inside that little cavity, which then translated for me: a claustrophobic experience!

As I approached the MRI machine, I assured the radiologist that I would probably meditate to keep my claustrophobia at bay. He said that ordinarily, the doctors gave their patients a tranquilizer. Hadn't I had one?

No.

He went on to say they knocked out children completely for the test. He said the noise frightened some people, but it didn't last. Each series of sound would be followed by a moment of silence while he readjusted the machine. The intervals of noise would last for seven minutes, twelve minutes, four minutes, up to forty-five minutes or an hour.

I figured I could handle it if I kept my eyes shut and meditated. I would not look at how much room I had once I was inside, and I would breathe steadily.

Bumpdebumpdebumpdebumpde. I was inside the sound with my eyes squeezed shut. I let my breathing and my mantra match with the machine's sound. I could handle this.

Clackclackclackclackclack. The new sound immediately shattered my rhythm into hundreds of tiny glass shards. When the high-pitched clacking stopped abruptly, I heard only my panting and heartbeat.

The radiologist's voice came into my strange sound space from a million miles away, "Are you all right?"

"Mmmmmmhuh," I said, not convincing either of us.

What else was there to do? I had to not move even a fraction of an inch because he had carefully measured my body before sliding me into the hole. My cooperation was essential to the success of taking these pictures of my spine, and they were vital to me. I had to see for myself what was happening inside, for I no longer trusted medical authorities to know what was best for me. I did not move, kept my eyes closed, concentrated on my mantra, and kept breathing, praying for the time to pass quickly.

Whhhhhhhhhhhhrrrrrrrr. Clacketyclacketyclackety. And on and on and on with occasional moments of an eerie silence, then the voice from a million miles away asking me how I was doing.

An hour and fifteen minutes later, I sat in the waiting room, dressed as the same person I had been before the MRI, but I felt like no one in particular. I felt stripped of something, not quite naked, but without some part of me. Though I thumbed through a magazine rather normally while I waited for the films, I was far from myself. Had the torturous sounds chased my soul away? Had the magnetic field fuzzed up my own electromagnetic field or blown it to bits? I felt dazed and distant, but pleased to have the films finally handed over to me. I would be the first to see them, which seemed only proper. My doctor had requested that I bring the films to my appointment on Monday. Rather than depend on the lab to deliver over the weekend, I took them home with me. I would have the whole weekend to study what I looked like on the inside.

When I arrived home, I opened up the large folder and pulled out fourteen photos, about fourteen by seventeen inches in dimension, showing my spine and cross-sectional views of the damaged disc. How was such a phenomenon possible? No longer immersed in the torture of it, I was suddenly awestruck by the technology that made it possible to see exactly what the inside of my vertebrae and discs looked like. My herniated disc, between the fourth and fifth lumbar vertebrae, was flattened and spilling pitifully out from all sides. I cried, noticing how dark and injured it seemed in the midst of the other healthy white discs above it. The discs below did not look all that great, but they were not spilling out. They were somewhat flattened and darker than the ones above. The cross-sectional views were a mystery. I would have to let my doctor decipher them. The only obvious fact was *subluxation* (misalignment) of the vertebrae on either side of the injured disc. I wondered if that had eventually caused the disc to herniate.

My partner wanted to hold me close after studying the films with me, but I still had that strange, stripped feeling and could not be touched yet. I thought standing next to the gnarly, forty-year-old weeping willow down the street from our house might help restore me. Though it was 10:00 P.M., we walked to the tree together, remembering the lounging raccoon family we had seen peering down at us through their little bandit masks the last time we had been there. I leaned the front of my body against the strong old willow, resting my cheek on its rough, furrowed bark, and tried to reach my arms around the trunk. I could only reach halfway around this giant tree with my arm span of six feet. I turned my body front to back and round again, imagining that the energy of the tree might help me knit back the electromagnetic field of my body, which seemed shattered by the MRI.

I wondered if there were any studies on the affects of the MRI on the electromagnetic field of the human body. I knew that mine had been seriously affected, that I needed to do whatever I could about restoring it. Since there were no facts on this, I would simply trust my intuition. I had a feeling the medical profession would not be interested in my response to the MRI. Still, I had a strong desire to let all patients who go through a Magnetic Resonating experience know that a restoration process was vital to consider in any way they chose.

After being with the weeping willow, I wanted to be near running water, which seemed impossible at that time of night. I settled for a warm bath and only then felt ready to be held by my partner, finally.

The next morning, I had physical therapy before meeting with my clients. I brought the MRI films to share with all the physical therapists. They crowded around the illuminating lamp, fascinated by what the MRI could show. I wondered why therapists did not have more opportunities to see what the doctors routinely observed, particularly since they did most of the work with their patients.

On Monday I met with my doctor to hear his translation of the films. I waited in the examining room for about twenty minutes while I heard him talking on the phone outside my door. I stopped being irritated about having to wait when I realized he was talking to the radiologist who interpreted my films. I began to tremble ever so slightly. Why were they taking so long in discussion before talking to me? What was wrong? The doctor finally came in and snapped on the illuminating light for x-rays so we could look at the films together. He said the herniated disc was pushing up against two nerve roots where they were attached to each other, making surgery not viable, and likely causing the severe symptoms I was having.

What made them attach? He said I was born this way, and

49

went on to explain that a congenitally joined nerve root is not necessarily serious in and of itself, nor is a herniated disc. As a matter of fact, he had seen worse discs with no symptoms. The specific problem for me was that my joined nerve root was unfortunate enough to be exactly where the herniated disc pressed, which aggravated the pain in the sciatic nerve running down my left leg. He showed me how this was happening on one of the cross-sectional views of the disc. He then showed me the deterioration in progress with the two discs below the injured one. Why was this happening? Questions tumbled out.

How could I stop the inflammation if every time I sat down, the disc bulged against the conjoined nerve root? Wasn't that what caused the inflammation in the first place? Yes, but the anti-inflammatory drugs and the physical therapy will help reduce it. But won't it come back again whenever I sit down? I remembered the graphs and photos I had seen in my back education class during physical therapy. Some very brave but crazy college students had volunteered for a study on the amount of pressure their discs withstood through sitting, standing, lying down, and lifting. Needles had been inserted into the center of each disc to record measurements. Thanks to them, I learned that sitting increased pressure by 150 percent over standing. Should I stop sitting altogether? That seemed to be the only variable within my control. I could do nothing about the joined nerve roots, and little about the natural wear and tear of aging.

My doctor told me not to make too much of the joined nerves because he believed that with time the disc would scar over and no longer press on the nerves. How long did that take? He explained that it was a slow process, since discs consisted mostly of cartilage. Anywhere from a year to two. He asked me how long I could sit now before I had tingling in my left leg. I estimated between fifteen and twenty minutes. He suggested that I get up and move around whenever I felt the nervy sensation in my leg, and definitely not sit beyond that time. Why was surgery not necessary? Because of the conjoined nerves, he did not want to risk more problems with the potential of surgically touching two nerves instead of one. If it had been only one nerve strand, he could more easily have moved around it to get to the disc.

He still believed the cortisone might eventually work in reducing the swelling of the nerve root. It could take up to ten days for any relief. In the meantime he wanted to check the weakness again in my left leg. After he performed the tests, we both agreed that my left toe seemed to hold a little longer than before, and so did my left foot when he pressed down on it. Though my left leg was still profoundly weaker than my right, possibly the strength was returning slowly but surely after the epidural. He reminded me that my sitting time had also increased from zero (I'd been feeling "nervy" immediately upon sitting down) to fifteen minutes after two months of healing. This was progress, albeit almost immeasurable. I left the office, trying my best to feel heartened and hopeful, with another two months' prescription for physical therapy. I was encouraged to keep walking, as it was one of the best exercises for strengthening all the muscles that would help hold my spine in its newly compromised position. It would simply take time.

I was very lucky to have a medical doctor who had faith in my body's ability to readjust itself and heal on its own without too much intervention from the outside. Though I had lost some confidence in both of us during the time my left leg muscles weakened so drastically, I was relieved to learn that surgery was not a viable option for me. This fact motivated me even more to walk myself back to health, and my clients benefited from my resurgence of faith in the natural healing process. I began to understand what my consulting analyst had meant when he said that it was a rare opportunity for clients to see how a healer approached her own healing, that such a witnessing process did not have to be burdening, but could be inspiring for clients.

What I noticed immediately with the people I walked with during that week was an increase in their self-confidence. It was clear to me that we shared an interactive field in which we influenced one another to the positive and to the negative, like all people who are connected to one another do. When we shared a bond, whether as client and therapist, friends or relatives, it was not just how we tended the other that made the impact on him or her, it was also how we tended ourselves.

In this, I realized I had even more of a responsibility than to myself as I continued to tap into the natural healing process available within the life force. Trees inspired me, and I inspired my clients. The gift economy worked easily when the joy of discovery was passed along. Whether or not we walked or sat together in the office, we shared an interactive field that served as a kind of invisible crucible in which creative and collaborative ideas flowed together to inspire healing. Our shared stories were support and nourishment for the journey.

CHAPTER 5

Sacred Collaboration

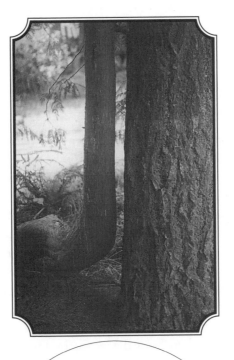

Sacred Collaboration

is demonstrated by a hemlock and pine

that grow in a co-housing community in Langley, Washington.

The younger tree started out life

at an angle that was guided back to an upright position by the

presence of the older tree. Growing side by side,

they now form with their upper branches the shape of a whole tree.

Chapter 5

Thea's smile radiated all through the depths of her wide-set green eyes. She put her hand straight out to shake mine and said, "I'm so glad to be here." Looking around my office, she considered which chair to sit in: a modernistic leather chair from Scandinavia or an old, soft chair in which she could sink into the pillows. She chose the soft one and cuddled back into it, but her feet did not touch the floor, so she moved forward and sat up straight. Thea wanted to understand the dreams that flooded her sleep time, becoming a world unto themselves she gladly stepped into at the end of each day. Her physical health was severely compromised with diabetes and intermittently recurring brain hemorrhages that had been diagnosed by the Mayo Clinic as untreatable beyond pain management. Walking therapy was not a possibility for us.

Also a writer who had published extensively over the last twenty years, Thea had founded a writing organization in her hometown. She and her husband had raised a son together while also providing a place in their home for her mother, who had Alzheimer's disease. A chore person came daily to take care of the mother's physical needs and to help Thea with any extra household work she was not able to manage herself. Though her life had changed drastically, she did not consider herself unable to live a meaningful life for as long as she could. Having recently participated in a writers' conference in which she was inspired by a dream workshop taught by one of my colleagues, Thea asked him for a referral to help her address her dreams and their relationship to her creativity. He had referred her to me, thinking I would be able to meet her more fully as both writer and psychotherapist.

Though she had not intended to begin psychotherapy, Thea felt certain that her dreams and her writing were connected in a mysterious way, and if that were true, she wanted to do her best by both of them. I had sent her a copy of my philosophy statement as an introduction to the kind of psychotherapy I practiced, letting her know that I worked with individuals and couples interested in personal and spiritual growth, understanding conscious and unconscious aspects of the self, healing, and creativity, as well as developing healthy relationships with others; that my specialization was in listening to and working with the creative process, a process I believed was natural and inborn; that I practiced a variety of interactive methods including voice-dialogue, dream work, active imagination, and sand-play; and when weather permitted, I walked with clients who wanted to combine dialogue, movement, and connection to nature as part of their healing.

Having stated and heard each other's intentions during our first session together, Thea and I met in my office once a week for an hour. Within four months I came to understand that what Thea and I were doing together was far beyond either of our statements to one another, and most likely beyond what I could articulate to anyone else except through story. It was true that she brought in her dreams and her writings, but she was also bringing in her life story; her devastatingly injured physical self; her past, present, and future; her hopes, disappointments, regrets; her humor and curiosity; her fresh intelligence, surrealistic imagination, and grief; her paintings, and failures; her shame; her childhood memories of parents and siblings, homes and friends; her unique angle on life and also on death.

Thea and I opened our hearts to one another. She was the

teller of her story, and I was the listener, both of which required our being present without any preconceived ideas about what was supposed to happen. We wanted to honor and let thrive whatever evolved spontaneously between us during our sessions. What this required of me was to do as Carl Jung suggested and leave my psychological textbooks, consultations, and my know-ingness outside the door of the therapy room. When encounter-ing the person who had come to be with me, what was most essential was to really be there in the present with them and with myself, open to see and hear what was actually so in the moment. When this was possible, something new emerged between us, something that could not have been known before.

Such witnessing required what James Hillman, Jungian ana-lyst, described as *notitia, the paying attention to the qualities of things as a primary activity of the soul. Notitia* was a Latin word conjugated from the root, *noscere*, meaning "to come to know," which suggested that what was noticed was not already known. Children practice *notitia* as a way of being. When infants discover a flower for the first time, they study the shape and colors, the way it moves, how it sounds, and the way it smells. All their senses are tuned to noticing the quality of each new being in their world. They want to interact and will likely wrap their tiny hands around a flower, sooner or later, to have a taste of it. Their hearts and minds are open, and their desire is to come to know what is in their lives by deeply noticing the quality of things.

Thea and I practiced noticing together with as little refer-ence to traditional psychotherapy as we could both tolerate. During our sessions I not only listened to her feelings and con-cerns, her stories and dreams; I also interacted and related to them and to her, paying close attention to what Aristotle called the *correspondences between things.* I discovered that there was an interactional field between us that had a life of its own and was beyond our consciousness. The closest I could come to describ-ing this field was to say that it was comparable to the creative space between writer and story, sculpture and stone, dancer and music—pairs that deeply affect one another, with neither half being solely responsible for outcome of their collaborative encounter, a relationship that is invisible but highly charged with possibility and new life.

Thea would tell me a dream which we tended together with care and concern; then she would come in the next week with a series of paintings that expressed her own interactions with another dream. We related to the dreams and paintings, noticing correspondences between the two, which would be followed by more, all of which became part of the interactional field between us.

We were in a creative process that neither of us could claim as our own, although it was composed of all that we brought to each moment we shared. There was a flow, a dynamic energy moving within and between us, both consciously and unconsciously, like a dance of spirits, no matter the content of our conversations. What I had learned through my own healing process became available to Thea in this field, whether or not I said anything about it, because this energy did not belong to me. It was a mysterious and unknowable force that lived in the space between us.

One of our sessions in particular revealed this phenomenon to me in a most poignant way through a story Thea told. She had been deeply moved by an experience she had after a previous session, when she had gone to the University Hospital for an MRI. This was something she had done routinely for the last several years to monitor the progression of her disease. Ordinarily, she would just drive home afterward, but this time she did not feel like getting in the car right away. Instead, she wandered over to another section in the hospital to see the displayed art work left by patients who had been or were still going through treatment for breast cancer. For some reason, unbeknownst to her, she still did not feel like driving home right away. But she did not know what else to do and wandered out to the parking lot. Noticing how beautiful the fall leaves were, she meandered over to the trees on the hillside behind the lot.

In telling me the story, Thea kept interrupting herself to say this behavior was very unusual for her and that her husband and stepson were rolling their eyes when she had told them what happened. She felt somehow invited over to a particular tree, so she followed the urge and thought she might just sit down and rest under it for awhile. Thea reached into her purse and said, "I brought this to show to you. Though it might seem like an old leaf, it really is something special to me."

I held it and turned it around, not recognizing the shape of the leaf that was as big as my hand. I admired the varied and golden tones of this leaf, which was predominantly rectangular but had two peaks at the top, on the left and right sides.

Thea said, "I don't usually do this kind of thing, but for some reason I thought, Oh, what the heck, why not? So I brushed off a spot to sit down, and I thought I'd try a little meditation. You know, just to see." She laughed nervously, almost apologetically.

But I could sense the excitement that was behind what she was about to reveal. I could also feel my own excitement rising to join hers, for I, too, had experienced a bit of an epiphany with a tree after my MRI.

"You won't believe this, Susan, but when I brushed off a place to sit down, there was this plaque. Right where I was going to sit!" She indicated the size with both hands, measuring about twelve inches long, maybe six to eight inches in width. "Here's what the plaque said." Reaching into her purse again she pulled out a scrap of notebook paper, put on her glasses, and read to me the story on the plaque. A physician had donated the tree to the hospital as inspiration for healing. It was a direct descendant of the plank tree that Hippocrates had sat under when he wrote the Hippocratic oath.

When she looked up, Thea had tears in her eyes. "When I sat there, I felt like Hippocrates was right beside me. Do you think that's possible?" She brushed her hair back, then pulled a Kleenex from the box beside her chair. "I mean not really, of course, but I had a real feeling of being connected through time.

I could picture him sitting under his tree, writing, just like I was." Then she laughed, "But I was just writing what was on the plaque. He was creating the Hippocratic oath!"

I reminded Thea that she had followed an unknown urge within herself to take a time out from her routine and go to the tree. I encouraged her to continue honoring such urges, and spend time under that particular tree as often as she could. She only needed to tend to whatever she noticed with fresh eyes within herself and outside as well. If she wanted to bring pen and paper to write or draw, I suggested she do so, but not as a chore. After all, Hippocrates had not known that what he recorded under his plank tree would endure over the centuries. He was only musing about what interested him most, deeply noticing the quality of things.

When Thea left, I found I needed time for taking note of what had just happened between us, via the spirit of Hippocrates, MRIs, and the inspiration of trees. My body wanted to move with all of it, so I walked the route near my office where I practiced walking therapy with my clients. Left foot, right foot, crunching through the fall leaves on the sidewalk. Lake Union on my left, blue sky overhead framed by the luminous gold autumn of trees lining the walkway. I felt grateful, reveling in the feelings cascading through me. The mysterious process of healing had just revealed a miraculous moment for both of us. Thea may have felt the moment differently, but feeling the same was not the essential ingredient between us, or within us. Something new had been born in our work together, and we would both be practicing notitia to see if we might come to understand it better.

I realized that psychotherapy was a creative process when not confined to being only a preconceived science. What was created in those moments had a little of every person in it, could not be owned by anyone, was part of the creative field, and included inspiration from past, present, and future. When such moments were related to with preconceived notions, no matter how positive such notions might be, what was beyond the frame likely would not be noticed or given a response. If, for example, I had shared with Thea what I already knew about archetypes and the symbolic meaning of trees throughout history, we would have missed experiencing the spontaneity of discovery, the authenticity of her own healing moment that was linked through time with Hippocrates.

Parenting can also be a creative process. In the past, parents who followed the principles of Spock were encouraged to be good parents by behaving in prescribed ways with their children. This was certainly helpful to many new parents who were frantic to do their best, but such a devotion to doing it right often precluded parents' learning from the child how to best respond to the child's self and her unique needs. An interactional field of mutuality and love must be present between parent and child in order for them both to grow into new aspects of themselves. Thea and I had related to each other from our different roles as client and therapist, yet neither of us needed to dominate, control, or already know before coming to know the quality of what was being discovered and shared between us.

We also needed to sustain our roles with each other in order for the magnetic field to be alive, as it was when there were two different poles. We could not have reversed roles or stepped out of the safe temenos we had created for our work together; nor could we have shared the same role, because the energy would have been repellent. For the creative flow to happen, as in a magnetic field, there must be two distinct poles. There had to be room between us for two with authority, not just one with authority, as can be the case in some models of psychotherapy in which control and behavior management are valued more than a client's discovery process.

During the next session Thea described an auto-driving excursion she had taken with her husband after her last brain hemorrhage. She had despaired over being housebound again and having to sit quietly or sleep for the next month while the blood leakage in her brain was reabsorbed. They decided to drive over the mountain pass and across the rolling prairies and farmlands of Eastern Washington into what is called the Tri Cities. She wanted to revisit her first childhood home, where she recalled fond memories of being age four, with her father, while he was tending his greenhouse. Thea remembered walking with him hand in hand into the humid, flowery air of the greenhouse, breathing deeply and looking around in amazement at all the colors. She would help him open or close the vents, whichever was called for, to keep the temperature and humidity just right for his cherished plants. As Thea spoke her eyes grew teary at the memory of these moments with her father.

She described other memories as well, of how most of her relatives were involved with the growing season in one way or another. Her mother canned fruit and vegetables for the family at harvest time, and during the growing season her uncle flew a crop duster plane over the surrounding fields. When they heard his plane flying overhead, Thea told me how she and her brother would race outside laughing and waving their arms, begging him to dust them, too. Waggling his wings first, he would then swoop low over the house and release the powdery yellow dust, covering them from head to toe.

61

"This was before we knew about the damage of DDT," Thea said, as a matter of fact.

I gasped.

She nodded seriously. "I talked to my Dad about all this before he died two years ago, and he felt really bad about it. We all wonder if it has something to do with what's happening in my brain now. But, you know, my brother's okay. Nothing wrong with him, or my sister either. So there's no way of knowing, and what difference would it make now? Probably no worse than just living there, downwind from Hanford."

Thea's childhood home in the Tri-Cities was an area known for a higher-than-normal percentage of mysterious health hazards. The nuclear reactor at Hanford had been shut down because of leakage into the environment, both airborne and through the water table. Anyone living in the area downwind from Hanford was known to be at a higher-than-normal risk for leukemia, birth defects, thyroid cancer, and many other forms of cancer in both the human and animal population.

Thea said, "Yeah, we're called the 'downwinders.' What a claim to fame."

Thea wanted to go on with her story of the driving excursion with her husband. She said nothing looked the same to her, that so much of what had once been expansive farmland was now suburbs or city buildings, cement and asphalt everywhere. She recognized none of the old landmarks as she approached her childhood home, causing her to wonder why she had embarked on such a journey after all. The countryside had evolved into a nondescript neighborhood just like any other. Thea thought she may as well have stayed in Seattle and driven around suburbs, which were more interesting aesthetically.

When they finally reached her childhood home, Thea recognized the shape of her father's greenhouse dilapidated beyond repair, but still standing. The sight of it overwhelmed her with joyful memories, losses, tears, a myriad of scents and sights, and deep longings she could not even name. She and her husband noticed the rusty sagging structure no longer had any windowpanes, though it still housed tables and pots that were now decayed and covered with weeds and trash.

Breaking through what used to be the glass ceiling of the green house, but which now was only a bent network of metal struts, stretched the topmost branches of a tree! Thea laughed in amazement. The tree's roots had cracked its own pot and grown through the floorboards into the earth. It was likely thirty-five years old by now, since that was how long ago her father had sold their property. Thea and her husband stood and stared for quite awhile before continuing on with their driving excursion. The sight of the tree breaking through its own house lifted enough of the despair Thea had felt following the latest recurrence of her illness that hope for her own life was restored. She returned home inspired to write again.

Different Rhythms

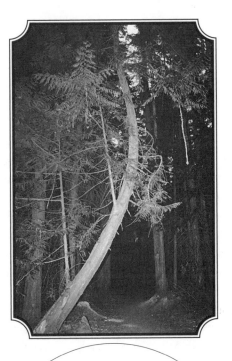

Different Rhythms *leaned,*

then turned toward light created by a trail cut into the forest

behind the high school on

South Whidbey Island, Washington.

Not only has it found its unique place in the sun, but this cedar has

also transformed two branches into trunks.

Chapter 6

When Jack, with whom I had worked on a weekly basis for over a year, decided to do walking therapy, I noticed immediately how expressive he was with his whole body, gesturing with arms and hands boldly to make a point. In the office he rarely moved at all.

In fact, he had seemed depressed, because the only emotion he consistently shared in the office was a quiet sadness, his hands motionless in his lap. Whenever he tried to access other feelings—anger in particular—he experienced so much shame he would remain collapsed in his chair. Until we walked, I had no idea that such constriction had to do with how he had been adapting his own body to the chair in the office. It had helped him sit on his feelings, to be out of rhythm with what was happening inside. His frustration, as well as excitement and enthusiasm, could finally emerge naturally and easily when we walked and talked because the emotional intensity and body motion matched up. Jack's emotional depth and complexity could be witnessed, experienced, and honored as we walked because of his obvious congruence.

I wondered how the practice of psychotherapy had developed over the years with such an enduring devotion for sitting, with no regard for the natural rhythms of our bodies. The stories shared in psychotherapy break hearts, infuriate us, and ignite despair, laughter, waves of peace and joy, deep curiosity, love, resentments. They cover the diverse range of emotions that make our hearts beat fast, our breathing quicken, the adrenaline flood through our bodies. Until my clients and I practiced walking together, we responded to all of it by sitting face-to-face, motionless in the chair. This could not be good for our bodies over time to be so incongruent with our basic life rhythms.

When Diana brought her six-month-old child Bridget into session, we sat in our usual talking positions, face-to-face, until Bridget wanted to crawl and explore the toy shelf. It felt quite natural to move from our chairs onto the floor to join the baby, while we continued to talk. Since the issues Diana was most concerned about had to do with motherhood and learning how to respond best to her daughter's needs, it made sense to include Bridget in our sessions. We tended easily to whatever her baby needed without feeling interrupted because Bridget was indeed an essential part of our therapy sessions. She even moved us outside to walk together, when she could not be consoled in the office.

Diana said, "I think she's just tired but can't relax enough to nap. Being in motion helps a lot. When I put her in the backpack and walk around the block, she's out like a light. Works every time."

By the time we had bundled her up—and ourselves as well—Bridget was already quiet and looking forward to our outdoor adventure together. Thus began walking therapy on a regular basis. Occasionally, Diana brought the stroller instead of the backpack, especially as Bridget grew heavier and more active. We took turns pushing the stroller, all the while walking and talking about motherhood, babies, and juggling time for self, husband, and creativity.

It was not the content of our conversations that made the difference in Diana's therapy, she told me later. The shared rhythms, camaraderie, and fresh air made her think better, made it possible for her to make more meaningful connections between past and present, and to feel less judgmental of herself or others. She thought it might have something to do with our actual physical movement. I agreed that walking side by side, rather than sitting face-to-face in the office, did open up the possibilities. We focused less on problems and pathologies and more on how things flowed or stopped. Our therapy itself seemed more in the rhythm of life when we walked and talked, pushing the stroller with a baby who not only was included in our therapy sessions but often guided them.

Some rhythms, though, called for staying in the office to tend in a more imaginative way the connection between humans and nature. I could not predict who might be more comfortable walking with me, and who needed a more cloistered environment for dealing with intimate subjects. I let each person decide what worked best and found that my clients began paying more attention to their own rhythms in anticipation of such choices as whether to stay in the office or walk and talk. Barry, a forty-five-year-old outdoorsman and field biologist, surprised me when he said he would not be comfortable being outside while talking about what he needed to address with me. We were working with his depression and fears of depression, as well as grief over his father's death the previous year. He had not been able to cry over the loss of his father, though he had mixed and complicated feelings that seemed impossible for him to express. This was a major complaint of his wife's. In their five-year marriage he had rarely been able to discuss emotions, though he was able to love, be supportive and present for her. Barry, an introverted, sensitive man, clearly had depth and passion to share, but was profoundly blocked from accessing and expressing it.

We met weekly in the office for seven months before he finally felt comfortable enough to try walking therapy. It began with a dream about his being flooded with tears, in danger of drowning. We both thought the dream had to do with his holding back feelings to the point of being completely overwhelmed by them. Before coming into therapy he had been involved with Alanon, a support group for family or friends of alcoholics. His father had died of chronic alcoholism, and he had learned that anyone who lived with or loved an alcoholic would benefit by treatment for codependence. Though there are many descriptions and behavior variations of codependence, the definition I prefer is the deferring of one's own truth. Barry found it most possible to be truthful with himself when he was alone in nature for long periods of time. His job as a field biologist was a perfect fit for him, but he found it difficult to maintain a sense of himself with others, particularly beloved others like his wife.

We had been focusing for the past few months in therapy on his learning how to maintain his own rhythms and how to keep his finger on the pulse of his emotions. In late June Barry strode happily into my office after spending three weeks in the mountains, suntanned and healthy, his smile peeking through a newly grown beard. Pleased with himself, he told me the story of calling his wife just before he went out on his latest job in the North Cascade Mountains. She had canceled a trip they had planned together in August for no apparent reason, other than she just did not feel like going. This made him angry, particularly since she had not considered how he might feel about it, not to mention she had made a unilateral decision. His first feeling was sadness, which he tried to hold to himself, but it slipped out anyway. Anger followed when his wife defended her own decision, and they got into an argument, which he felt bad about after hanging up the phone.

He proceeded with his day's work, thinking it best to work out his anger on the trail, then call her when he returned, but he ended up having to spend the night in the mountains. He felt almost desperate to call and make sure everything was okay between them, but gradually he gave up and thought of it as a forced exercise in working out his codependence. The next morning, he said he felt rewarded for his progress by finding a nest of spotted owl babies. He considered them to be a sign of the treasures in store when he finally is able to tell the truth about himself.

We celebrated this rite of passage with a handshake; then he leaned back in his chair and pondered in silence for a long while before telling me another story. His voice grew soft as he began to describe what else happened to him during the last three weeks.

"You know, I've always been at home outdoors, even as a kid. I'm cautious about things and alert, but most of the time I feel relaxed and strong in my own territory."

I nodded.

He carried himself with confidence and was definitely fit and able, six feet, two inches tall, probably 180 pounds. Barry looked down and almost whispered, "I used to love camping beside a roaring stream, but I can't anymore."

I waited for him to go on, but it took him a long time to speak again. He looked up and crossed his arms.

"They scare me when I get too close to them now."

I asked, "How long has this been going on?"

"Just this last time in the mountains. Maybe since that drowning dream a couple of weeks ago." He rubbed his beard and said, "You know I used to feel inspired and powerful beside a wild stream. It's so weird to try and stay away from them now."

"Maybe you could sit by some calmer ones to start with to see what occurs to you. Your dream was about drowning in tears. Perhaps it's time to be with your sadness."

He nodded. "Wouldn't it be great if something came of it all, like finding those owls?"

At the end of session I said, "Good luck with your stream-therapy."

He was delighted with the play on words, thinking at first I had said *dream-therapy.*

A month passed before Barry returned from the mountains. He had camped intentionally by a stream for two days and was not frightened the whole time, but the river had been low and calm due to the drought. He said there were plenty of roaring streams up where he was working, and he would eventually get close to them. Maybe next time out. I mentioned walking ther-apy as a possibility if he wanted to try and face the stream with my company. He seemed quite nervous about this idea, so I said he could let me know when and if he ever wanted to do walking therapy with me. In the meanwhile we would do our *stream* work from the office.

Barry brought his dream journal with him for the next session a week later. He wanted to tell me the dream he had about doing *stream-therapy* with me.

He read aloud, "Susan and I are driving our pickup trucks into the wilderness. We come to a pond, where we see a big bullfrog and the dorsal fins of carp swimming around. There's a house in the distance. We put our kayaks in and paddle around, splashing and playing like sea otter. We're having much fun together before eventually settling down to talk about stream-therapy. There's a woman on shore who's watching us. I say I'm afraid.

"Susan says, 'I haven't done this before and I don't know what's going to happen.'

"I laugh and say, 'If you did, you'd be charging a lot more money for this.'

"Susan starts telling me sad stories about her father dying and I begin to cry. I feel very sad for her and give her a hug for comfort, but I feel really awkward. The woman on shore shouts, 'Isn't it supposed to be the other way around?'

"Susan says to me, 'Since you are not connected to your sadness directly, I'm trying to help you find your tears this way.' End of dream."

I asked Barry what he thought of doing walking therapy with me, perhaps even crying in my presence. He said it sounded okay during last session, but then he started worrying about therapy outside the office and wondered if he would be able to do it right. He thought he might feel less self-conscious trying *stream-therapy* and crying completely by himself, then telling me about it later. I respected Barry's need to feel safe both in the new territory of walking therapy and in the new territory for him of intense emotion. I told him that the dream figure of the watching woman on shore was an important one for him. She

69

intended to protect him and was very certain about doing what was right for Barry. I was glad to see such a presence in his psychology, for she would be an ally in his struggle to stand up for his own truth and not defer to others.

Then I described what I had learned by walking with clients to date, that every session was different and based on what came up for each person, that I tried to respond without expectations, since I truly did not know what would come up. In that regard, his dream was right about my *not knowing what would happen*. Walking therapy was a completely new idea for me, not yet defined except by those who participated in it with me. I told Barry that it was about learning together in nature, that I found nature to be helpful in this discovery process, but that the basic integrity of the therapeutic relationship would always be honored, with or without walls. This meant that sessions would be an hour long, paid for at the same rate as in the office, not social meetings, but working sessions devoted to his healing process.

I explained that as was true with office therapy, walking therapy, too, could be playful and fun, serious, scary, sad, with all the feelings he had dreamed about. I assured him again that the watching woman on shore belonged in all therapies, and that we would always check in to make sure she understood and approved the process. I suggested we continue working with his water dreams, thus doing *stream-therapy* through active imagination in the office.

He said, "Sounds good to me. I have a couple more dreams to tell you, then: I'm going down a river and come to a big logjam. I fall into the water, injure my head, and can't talk for several weeks, but eventually I'm okay.

"Here's the next one." Putting the journal down, Barry looked up and smiled, "They seem kind of obvious now: I'm hiking with my wife and another couple. They want to set up camp in one place, but I really know of a better site. No one is listening to me, and I lose it. Suddenly I'm screaming and crying in front of everyone. I refuse to continue on in their direction.

Different Rhythms

They try to calm me down and talk me out of it, but I tell them to stop. I don't want consolation. I want my feelings. Then I cross a stream and my friends quietly follow me over to the other side. The site is better for everyone."

By summer's end, Barry had made an important decision to accept an advancement in his work, which would mean three months away from his wife, something to which she had always objected and to which he had deferred. This time he insisted, and she surprised him by agreeing to take a month off from her own job to join him in the field for a shared adventure. Before he left, Barry dreamed that I had invited him to a good-bye dinner to tell him that his dreams were his best friends. He had in fact learned to honor his own truth and rhythms, which eventually included self-initiated walking therapy in its own right time.

CHAPTER 7

Challenges

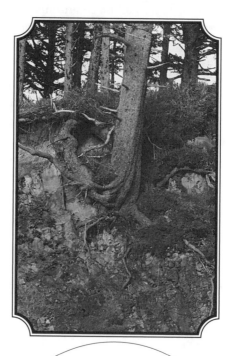

Courage *clings to the side of*
a cliff that has dropped away from under it.
By changing its
exposed roots into trunk cells
this tree has sustained and supported its continual growth
at the north end of Cannon Beach, Oregon.

Chapter 7

When my office building closed down for a month of renovations, I was faced with the decision again of taking off time from seeing clients, doing walking therapy with everyone, or renting office space from a colleague. I chose to sublease an office in the Fremont district of Seattle, where there was a path along the waterway connecting Lake Union with Puget Sound through a series of canal locks. Clients could choose their own rhythm for doing therapy: sitting in an office, walking with me in the Fremont neighborhood, or walking in the city parks. Catherine, a sixty-year-old woman who had recently returned from a writer's retreat in New Mexico, was ordinarily a calm, articulate, reflective, and spiritually attuned woman, but she came into my new office for her therapy session visibly agitated. She could hardly sit still in her chair, and she kept crossing and uncrossing her legs while trying to describe what had happened to her at the retreat.

"I don't know whether I'm more furious at myself or the writing instructor, or what," she said, leaning forward in her chair, about ready to jump out of her skin.

I nodded, suggesting she go ahead and stand up, move around the room.

Immediately she stood up and pounded her fist in her hand. "Oooh. I'm so mad," she said, pacing back and forth across the room. She tried to sit down again, but could not stay put. "Maybe we should walk. I'm too wound up to sit on all this."

As we walked side by side through a quiet residential section in Fremont, Catherine was finally able to tell the story of being shut down for the whole retreat. It had all started when her male instructor overtly and consistently gave preference to the younger students whose writing was modern and experimental, more like his own. She had finally gotten up enough nerve on the fourth day to ask for a private consultation on her manuscript, since she had been ignored in class. Her trepidation proved to be well-founded when she received a rejecting evaluation that not only dismissed her writing but also devalued her as a person, leaving her speechless and horrified.

Catherine had already felt self-conscious and out of place being the only grandmother in a class of predominantly twenty- and thirty-year-old students. Though she had written sporadically throughout most of her life, publishing magazine articles and short stories, she had not found enough time until her children left home to devote her creative energies to a novel. The last class in writing that Catherine had taken in college was too many years ago to count. She had hoped that by going to the retreat for encouragement and honest critique she might turn her beloved story into a novel. But she had returned from the retreat humiliated, diminished, completely blocked, and unable to write a word.

"What's wrong with me that I could let such a jerk collapse me like that?" Catherine's cheeks were flushed. "I couldn't say a word. I just sat there stunned stupid!" Her walking pace was fast and furious, hard to keep up with.

I smiled, happy that we could walk together through her fury. It was the first time in the six months we had worked together that I had witnessed anything but her gentle, thoughtful, very careful consideration of things. Now her passions spilled over the edge, flushing her face with a beautiful vitality.

"I've been such a pressure cooker. Ready to explode. I wish I could have said something, anything to that man. Oooh, it makes me so mad that I just sat there!"

Catching up with her, I puffed along beside, "What would you have said, Catherine?"

Without a moment's hesitation she said, "You can't hold me back. I've already had the brakes on for too long. Move out of my way, now." She added in almost a whisper, "You pompous ass." Then she took a deep breath and said with resignation, "Oh, Susan, I can't do it. He's not here. It's too late, anyway." Her boiling rage bubbled down to a simmer, then suddenly dropped her into sorrow, and finally into tears.

"Well, he might be here, after all," I said. "At least someone like him not too far from here. It would mean adding a half hour to our session and a walk up to the top of that hill." I pointed across the street. "I'm willing if you are."

Wiping the tears away, Catherine said, "Maybe. What are you talking about?"

We stopped in the middle of the sidewalk to make our decision about whether to return or extend the session for another half hour. Ordinarily, I required advance notice to schedule extra time, but I did not have an appointment after Catherine's. Not only was there time now, but she needed support in that particular moment to find her voice. I described the Fremont Troll rising up from the mud under the Aurora bridge. Several years previously, a group of artists in the community had joined together to build a twenty-foot-high concrete sculpture of a one-eyed troll, whose gnarly hand covered a life-size Volkswagen. Though everyone, adult and child alike, knew it was not alive, primitive feelings always emerged whenever they confronted the troll. Since we were close to its neighborhood, I thought we might make a visit and see what happened when she had support in facing an actual monster. I did not think it mattered whether or not the troll symbolized a person in her life or whether it represented an energy residing within her own self.

When we arrived at the base of the sculpture towering above us, Catherine studied the troll in minute detail for close to ten minutes in awestruck silence. Finally, she moved close enough to its huge hand to touch the knuckles, then around to each side to see its profile. Cautiously, she peeked inside the Volkswagen. Her feelings came forth as she imagined herself in the car, having just been snatched from the bridge above and derailed from her rightful path. Catherine pictured the darkness and feelings of suffocation she might have if she were actually inside the Volkswagen, not able to get out because of the troll's grip on her.

Rage at the writing instructor paled in light of the dawning awareness that she had been blindly following an *internal script* for most of her life, one that reined her in, held her down, kept her small. The writing instructor had blindly stepped into the role and played out this script in actuality, awakening Caroline to her rage. She alternated between tears and rage, pacing in front of the troll, feelings streaming from her. She moved from the essence of child to warrior to bereft woman who had lost too much time already to hold back any longer on her passions. She found the flow and rhythm of her voice that day as her body in motion took over and showed her how to let go of the old story and create a new one.

76

With walking therapy, creative challenges abounded. There

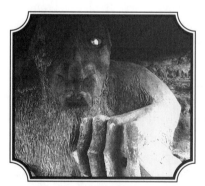

were no role models or guides to follow in doing psychotherapy outside, so my clients and I had to continuously adjust, adapt, and rely on our wits to tend with whatever came across our paths. In sharing such collaborations with one another, we were stepping into territory very different from most self-help or psychological models. We were not trying to fix or perfect ourselves; rather, we

Troll is a community sculpture that stands more than twenty feet tall under the Aurora Bridge in the Fremont area of Seattle. Though not a living tree, it has served as a touchstone to many who are familiar with the Billy Goats Gruff fable.

were changing our patterns of perceiving by noticing and interacting with what we discovered together in life outside the office. We were learning how to accept what was not perfect or well-developed in ourselves. Practicing psychotherapy outside the office allowed me opportunities to see my imperfections as a psychotherapist, to learn to forgive and change with each experience. We were all learning to traverse new territory, and the challenges were plentiful. How would I protect one of the time-honored tenets of psychotherapy, confidentiality, when we might run into friends while doing walking therapy together?

One of my clients, Molly, helped initiate us into facing this challenge openly, honestly, and with an instinctual firmness that emerged spontaneously during one of our walks. We had met in the parking lot of Discovery Park and congratulated ourselves for escaping the Blue Angels, which were currently flying directly over my office with earsplitting sonic booms. Since she had walked in this park before, I suggested she choose the trail.

She seemed surprised and said, "You mean you don't have a standard route that everyone goes on?"

I said, "We're pioneers, Molly. We'll have to find our path together."

She shrugged, "Well, okay, then."

As we headed uphill to the bluff trail, we agreed to check our watches in about half an hour, then return down the same route so our walk would be an hour long. About fifteen minutes into our session, friends of mine called out, waved, and moved toward us for a conversation. Quickly, I called back that I would talk with them another time and put up my hand in a stopping gesture. I had to walk right past them, wishing I had a sign on me that read, In Session. Do Not Disturb. But that would present a confidentiality problem. My friends were clearly surprised by my abruptness, but I could think of nothing else to do.

When my client and I arrived at the bluff, we stood for about ten minutes, talking about and gazing at the water, the Olympics beyond, the boats, and barges below. Molly said she felt peaceful, that usually she walked faster on her own just for the workout. Walking and talking with me slowed her down to a pace that changed the whole rhythm of her thinking process. She was not so intent on problem-solving within our hour of walking because she felt like there was more space and time to deal with things.

Happy to have reclaimed something she had known was an important part of her life but had literally forgotten up until our walking therapy together, she decided to put the activity on her calendar as a regular event. As a retired dancer, body movement had not found a natural next expression. She was choosing walking now. She told me she did not like to walk with most other people because there was so much conversation inside herself that another person tended to interrupt her thinking. During the next session, she told me she had walked in the park every day after work that week, ending at the bluff with the panoramic view of the sound at sunset. It had made all the difference in her week. Molly felt more confident that it might be possible to not *lose herself* to the demands of her job when she could honor her own rhythms better.

Most of my clients preferred choosing different walking therapy routes. Some liked to walk in the neighborhoods, while others preferred to schedule their sessions in one of three Seattle parks. Laurel preferred alternating time outside at Myrtle Edward Park with time inside the office. Her therapy focused on breaking the addictive patterns of a food-bingeing and purging cycle. Recently she had started a course of antidepressant medication that calmed her chronic anxiety. She'd been reporting a sense of feeling trapped, of being claustrophobic almost. She liked the open space of walking in the park with me, but also felt angry in the midst of her changing patterns. Because the antidepressant medication was taking away the edge, food no longer provided familiar relief. She was still left with the persecuting inner critical voice that wanted to purge her to perfection. This felt like torture without the occasional high she had gotten from bingeing. The addictive pattern was still strong within Laurel.

78

Challenges

She did not look well when she arrived for one of our walking sessions. Puffy and tired, clearly out of sorts, she said she was not doing well, that she had lied to her husband about having allergies instead of telling the truth about being hungover from a binge-purge cycle. She had to miss her nephew's baseball game, which she had been looking forward to all week, and was sad about how her addiction was taking her away from what she wanted. Away from life. Away from being outside like this, where she could breathe better. But her critical, condemning voice was also going wild with cynicism. She wanted to just block out the negativity and slow down her rhythms with something besides food-bingeing.

She hoped that walking might help change the rhythm of her thought process, that it might distract her from the critical inner voice for an hour, at least. I thought that our walking rhythm and what we might see together in the natural world had a good chance of interrupting her pattern of thinking, perhaps changing the brain waves. I asked her to notice if the purpose of her critic might be to protect her from being too vulnerable. But, by closing her down, it ended up being a persecutor, not protector. If we could help her find a more reliable way to open up and close down her vulnerability by choice, perhaps the critic would not do it with sarcasm.

Before the next session Laurel called to reschedule our time for the office. She arrived with a wrapped box and some drawings and asked to sit on the floor. I moved my chair back to sit down with her. She placed all of her items between us, seemingly comfortable and relaxed. Excited about sharing her treasure box with me, Laurel opened it up to reveal photographs, and every single card and letter she had ever sent to her grandmother. Laurel's mother had found them saved and dated in a drawer after the grandmother's death in 1990. She thought Laurel might like to have her childhood letters back. Whenever Laurel needed a reminder that someone in her family loved her, she opened the box and sorted through what her grandmother had cherished of

Laurel's photos, cards, letters, and gifts. The act of her grand-mother's dating and laminating Laurel's childhood photos meant that she was highly valued, at least by her grandmother. While we looked through her box together, I enjoyed seeing Laurel far less critical of herself, seemingly more trusting of her own nature, as she imagined herself through her grandmother's eyes.

We met again at the park for the following session. Laurel reported that she was beginning to feel some odd sadness about how eating was losing its magic for her. We discussed the need to substitute program for food, and how she might need a transi-tional object to replace the loss. She mentioned her infant niece, who needed a *blankey*, or pacifier, to help her through the transition from nursing. In just that moment, we discovered a baby seal crawling up the beach on the left side of our path. Watching closely, Laurel told me how people are not to bother them, because often their mothers are hunting nearby. We both worried, though, that the mother might not come back because of all the people at the park. She said she would call the Humane Society right away and get the number of marine wildlife to protect the baby.

"I bet that baby wishes he had a blankey right now," Laurel said.

Later that day, I received a call with her update on the baby seal. It had been there for a month, a vet checked him daily, and they had tried to relocate him once, but he returned. He was healthy and gaining weight. Laurel suggested they put up a sign, so people would know what to do and especially what not to do when they discovered the baby on the beach. She said to me before hanging up, "I'll see you next Saturday and we'll check on the baby."

When she arrived for the following session, Laurel was resentful about having to awaken so early to meet me. Angry at me, but not exactly. She wanted to feel safe about being angry. She continued yelling a bit, which she said felt good since she never let herself do that in my office for fear of interrupting other clients in the building. We walked and talked, and I told her of my conversation with her eating disorder specialist. Laurel had been discharged from the hospital almost a year previously and had tried the support of Overeaters Anonymous and another eating disorder group. She told me about planning to get a complete physical with a new doctor who specialized in treatment for food addictions.

She cried, "I'm afraid to hope again, Susan."

As we walked past the beach, we both noticed the baby seal was not there. Laurel then told me a dream: She was traveling in a 1957 Chevy, feeling strong and happy. At the doctor's office, she accepted her own handicap as a midget. The doctor restrained her arms down at her sides while she gave birth to a healthy baby almost as big as she was. During the pushing she felt panicked, claustrophobic, and she wanted the doctor to release her arms, but he wouldn't until she delivered the baby. End of dream.

I thought Laurel's dream indicated a desire to go through her fears about giving birth to self. Her fear of suffering had blocked this birth in the past. Perhaps she was finally ready for this birth after her long decline. Accepting, rather than denying and fighting her handicap, she now felt more able to struggle through pain, though she still needed help to do so. We noticed the baby seal was swimming in the sound as we returned down the path past his beach, both of us feeling hopeful for the new life abounding inside and outside.

Not every experience in the outdoors evoked such synchronous moments as Laurel and the baby seal, though. Eric was a client who expressed no interest in doing therapy outside until we worked with his dream about a rose. He had felt ecstatic looking into the center of the rose in his dream, and wondered what it meant. I could imagine plenty of possibilities and so could he, but I thought it might help amplify the dream further to enact it with him. We scheduled our session for the rose garden near the Woodland Park Zoo to see what might evolve from following the dream's suggestion. Our modified experiment in walking therapy would have to do with strolling through the roses until Eric found the one he wanted to gaze into. Then, as witness, I would facilitate any further imagery or experiences that might come up.

A family emergency interrupted our plans by calling him away from town for several weeks. By the time we finally did meet in the garden, he was still upset over the family crisis. We focused mostly on his distress while the roses provided only background for our discussion. We sorted through the repetitive motif of issues that had persisted throughout his lifetime. These family dynamics were not likely to change no matter what he did, and I began to wonder if focusing on them had already taken too much of Eric's attention away from his own life.

Several days later, he called to leave a message on my voicemail asking if I thought he was doomed by having such a dysfunctional family as he had. I called back and talked him through his despair, reminding him that we still needed to see what his rose dream wanted us to understand. When I recounted the story to my consulting analyst, he suggested that I might have been overcome by his family too, which is why I had not been able to help Eric follow the gift of his dream. The roses themselves could have helped us, he said with a smile, if only we had turned toward them.

Fortunately, the dream image endured with Eric. A year later, at his wedding, long-stemmed red roses were given to all members of the newly joined families and friends who came to celebrate Eric and his wife and the love to which they had both opened their hearts.

Embracing All

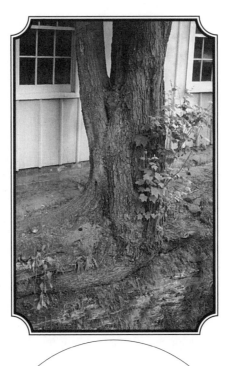

Embankment *grows along*
a stream running through Mount Holyoke College campus
in South Hadley, Massachusetts.
Its roots provide support for the bank while also nourishing
its trunk.

Chapter 8

Slowly but surely, my back became more stable with the support of physical therapy, walking, reduced sitting, and the support of both natural and allopathic medicine. After six months, though, I began to develop severe headaches that were occurring more and more frequently the better my back became. Was there a relationship? Nothing made the headaches go away—not abstaining from any foods, not massage, not drugs, not rest, or working out. I thought the headaches might be an expression of depression from being in chronic pain. I worked with my analyst and my dreams to see if this might be so, but nothing at the unconscious level was being revealed to me. Finally, I noticed that my headaches amplified intensely whenever I did my inverted back exercises, either on the traction board or on the physical therapy ball. Perhaps it had to do with the circulation of blood in my brain.

I consulted with a highly recommended homeopath and an osteopath, but concluded that my own instinct was the most reliable guide on how to integrate all that I had learned to date. The professional healers helped me select what I needed to know from each of my consultations without denying my own authority. So far, it had not been possible to *buy* any one system of thought in the healing of my back. I learned by keeping my finger on the pulse of the injury itself, not on what others believed about the healing of herniated lumbar discs and sciatic nerve radiculopathy. My injury had already sensitized me to many issues, not just my work with clients, but the whole idea of healing, authenticity, creativity, and how they were all interwoven.

While I continued to learn about my body and how it healed in compensatory ways, very much like the trees I observed, I noticed that my lower back had lost its curve. I wondered if the lack of curve had caused the degenerating spine or vice versa. The spine naturally curved in two places to cushion the weight of the head and torso: The cervical curve was at the neck and the lumbar curve at the lower back. What happened to the whole spine when one of the curves straightened out? I tried to apply to myself what I had learned from noticing how trees compensated by distributing weight and branches to balance themselves. Experimenting with my own body's trunk, I could feel immediately what happened to the cervical curve when I completely straightened the lumbar section of my spine.

I showed my spine doctor what I had discovered about this simple compensation on his plastic model of the human spine. When I straightened the lumbar portion of the spine, the model naturally thrust its neck forward. I asked if this might be causing my headaches. Perhaps the weight of my head thrusting forward like that was putting too much pressure on my cervical discs, thus creating the unrelenting headache pain. Already I had learned in physical therapy to lift objects close to my body because the weight-pressure increased incrementally as a law of physics when held away from the body. When my head's weight was carried at the top of my spine rather than at a forward angle to my body, the discs would bear the weight they were designed to bear. In focusing only on the healing of my lower back, had I inadvertently caused damage to the cervical discs?

Sadly, x-rays proved this to be true. As in my lower back, the pivotal disc at the center of the curve in my neck also looked like a flat tire. The disc material had not herniated or bulged against the spinal nerve, much to my great relief. My doctor said flattened discs were a typical part of the aging process, that there was nothing to do about it, but stay healthy and fit. He explained that everyone shrunk in height as they aged, since their discs eventually wore out, just like shocks on a car. I wondered how this would translate with the trees. I sensed they would find ways to compensate with new life somewhere else, or they would change shape to rely on another stronger part, until it was time to die. Then they would provide nourishment for the new life to follow.

When I left my doctor's office that day, I made a point of tucking my chin to relax my neck curve into its proper place without letting it thrust my head forward. My physical therapy now included care and treatment of the whole spine, rather than just focusing on the injured areas. Within a very short time, my headaches miraculously disappeared. I had finally learned to embrace the healing of my whole spine, not just a part of it. At least in that moment. I recognized that such a practice would be a lifetime devotional. I had been lucky enough to literally experience how to follow my instincts into new curves of my life. This eventually meant applying what I had been learning through nature to all my relationships, not just with clients. How to discover with beginner's eyes what was happening in life with my partner, friends, family, clients, and colleagues, not to mention myself. Nature, by way of the lives of trees, had opened this gift of different vision in me, as well as a desire to share with others what I was beginning to see. I began to take written note of the stories that sprang forth.

As writer, psychotherapist, and stepparent of five children, I had tried to balance my life so my three devotions would have an equitable share of my time. Though I was not always successful with this juggling act, I tried to write three mornings per week no matter what else called to me. Nature guided me to what wanted to be voiced and inspired me when I was depleted. Before, during, and after writing time, I found replenishment, whether I was walking in the woods or sitting in my backyard watching the sky. When I let myself be moved by the shape and texture of a particular tree, when I felt awed by the way it had found to grow in spite of obstacles, or sometimes because of certain obstacles, when I sensed myself pulsing with emotion as I stood next to such a magnificent, gnarled piece of life, I realized I felt love. Regeneration always followed, and soon I was writing again from an even deeper place in myself.

I found myself questioning, through my writing, what the practice of walking therapy was all about. I still wondered if walking might be a seasonal adjunct to what I did the rest of the time; thus, would I need to invest in a good ergonomic sitting chair for the coming winter? Or, was my back injury and the resulting changes in my work and my life an opportunity to create something new, something that had wanted to be born all along but had not been allowed before I was cracked open to another way? I wanted to keep my eye on the more judgmental part of myself who considered walking therapy to be an adjunct, as if it were dependent or subordinate to regular therapy. On the other hand, if I were to remain true to the original gift of the tall cedar with new life growing from its burl, I would have to concede that new life was profoundly related to the old. I would stay open to noticing what was so over time. For all I knew, maybe it was the other way around—that office therapy had evolved from the natural practice of walking and talking that beckoned us as far back as days of Plato and Socrates.

Tentatively at first, I began to share with a few friends what I was learning from nature. Since I was traversing the territory between two worlds, I did not yet have a language that could translate what happened in this space. I relied on my camera for awhile but found the language of photographic image to be just as limited as my written descriptions. My words represented the human world, and the photos tried to represent nature, but what would represent the space between? What was I learning about the interaction between past and present? Though I felt more interested in the present, which chronic pain can keep one attuned to, I knew from reading the life stories of trees during my daily pilgrimages into nature that all of time mattered in the shaping of the life force.

Synchronicity, the coinciding of time, was a particular meditation of mine during one of my reflective writing mornings, when I received two phone calls from old friends I had not been in contact with for over a year. Both lived in San Francisco, and neither knew the other, and neither had heard the story of my struggle to heal from the herniated disc. After our conversations I felt that I must truly be part of a much larger interactional field than I had previously fathomed. One of my friends had just called to offer me a free companion trip airline ticket to London and asked if I would like to fly with her, business class, in two weeks. But I could not even imagine such a possibility. My friend, on the other hand, could not believe I needed even an extra minute to consider her generous offer. I hung up the phone and stretched my back flat on the porch to let the sun inspire me. I could only picture how difficult it would be to travel with a severe back injury. Carry luggage? Impossible. Sit on an airplane for ten hours? No way. I would not be able to walk after that. And what about finances? There was nothing extra to spend. I would have to say no.

At 10:00 AM the phone rang again. One of my writing colleagues had just called long-distance to say hello, realizing we had not been in touch for awhile. We talked for a long time about our lives and current events. Mine, of course, was mostly about my back and walking therapy. His stories focused on his recent marriage. I mentioned the call I had just received and how at any other time in my life I would have gladly received such a gift and adventure. After hearing me tell of how I had reluctantly declined the airline ticket because I could not travel with a back injury, he encouraged me to reconsider. Synchronistically, one of his part-time jobs was as a public relations director for a walking tour company based in England. He thought I might want to do one of their tours since walking was so clearly healing for me, and the tour company needed photojournalists. If I changed my mind about going to London, he would see if there was a walk scheduled through the countryside of England, in case I was willing to take photos and write about the trip. My way would be paid, if the public relations office could use my photos.

Bewildered by my sudden good fortune in the midst of such a difficult healing journey, I wondered what to make of it all. Thrilled with the possibility, but still unsure if traveling would be good for my back and my healing process, I needed to *sleep on* the idea before making a final decision. I also needed to be certain my clients would be covered by another therapist during my absence. I would only have two weeks to prepare for the trip. Could I be in good enough physical shape to endure the daily walking for a week? Where would I find the extra energy? Constant pain was immensely fatiguing and it never disappeared.

On the other hand, with a herniated disc, rebuilding the muscles surrounding the vertebrae and keeping them strong was essential. I already had learned the hard way that sitting, being stationary, was the worst possible treatment, so it did not take me long to realize that a week's worth of daily walking would be perfect. I said yes to both friends when we all discovered the timing coincided perfectly for both the London flight and the walking tour of the Cotswolds. Immediately, I put myself on a walking program around Green Lake with the hopes of building up to three miles in the morning and three miles in the evening by the time I left for San Francisco. I would have to develop some stamina to travel from Seattle to San Francisco to London to the Cotswolds and back, and to tramp through the countryside ten miles a day for a week.

After sending out a notice to clients of my scheduled time off in a few weeks, I dug out my hiking boots and lovingly saddle-soaped them. My first attempt at the walk around Green Lake was disappointing beyond scope. I could only take small steps without aggravating my back. Besides, my right knee swelled up, meaning that the hiking boots had to go. I tried again the next day with my high-top tennis shoes and made it all the way around in about ninety minutes—three times as long as usual—came home, put a bag of ice on my back, and fell asleep.

I dreamed that I was trying to decipher a complicated document that had tiny print and large musical notes on the pages. I did not know what to do with the document. Not only did I not have my glasses; I did not know how to read musical notes. I found a music studio and went inside to see if someone could show me how to decipher the text. After listening to the music and watching some people dance, I understood that I had to immerse myself in the rhythms to understand the text. When I awoke from this dream, I recognized it to be another pearl on the growing strand of synchronicities, revealing what was hidden from my ordinary viewpoint.

I felt that I needed to let myself relax into the rhythm of the force that was bearing me along on this odd pilgrimage. So far, I had been knocked from my therapist's chair to walk with my clients, then for my own healing, all the while noticing with beginner's eyes how nature healed and regenerated. Now I was being presented with a chance to walk with others in foreign territory, not as a wounded healer but as a fellow wayfarer who would be taking photos and writing of our common experience. I wondered if the dream message of immersing myself in the rhythms was as simple as living life to know it, in contrast to the studying and analysis required of most psychotherapies.

I recalled Jung's famous quote about how life itself was the best of all teachers:

Anyone who wants to know the human psyche
would be better advised to bid farewell to his study,
and wander with human heart through the world.
There, in the horrors of prisons, lunatic asylums and
hospitals, in drab suburban pubs, in brothels and
gambling halls, in the salons of the elegant, the
Stock Exchanges, Socialist meetings, churches,
revivalist gatherings, and ecstatic sects, through love

and hate, through the experience of passion in every
form in his own body, he would reap richer stores of
knowledge than textbooks a foot thick could give
him, and he will know how to doctor the sick with
real knowledge of the human soul.[1]

But the dream wanted me to immerse myself in the rhythms
to understand the texts, not necessarily leave all texts behind.
I did not think my dream suggested I leave my profession; rather,
I thought it meant I needed to change the way I did things.
Perhaps radically. Not analytically, but rhythmically. What were
all the synchronous moments revealing about what was clearly
before my eyes but not yet recognized? They were related to
movement in the natural world and looking closely at life in the
present. Perhaps this was a clue to bringing alive what was in the
texts, or very possibly it was what was missing from the texts. So
much of analytical psychology referred to ancient wisdom as if
the soul could be found only in the past, not the present. But my
experience of healing with nature revealed the extraordinary
wisdom of the life force in the present. I was learning to read
stories of the life all around me, where alchemy was not an
esoteric philosophy but a fact of life in its most natural rhythms
and cycles.

During our transatlantic flight I noticed through my window
the sun illuminating vast turquoise mountains of ice in the white
landscape below. Sunrise or sunset, I could not be certain. My
sense of time and direction was changing as we flew what seemed
to be counterclockwise with time, from San Francisco to
London. Blinking against the glare, I wondered how long I had
been dozing, whether we were above Iceland or the Arctic.
I savored the curious sensation of hovering in space like the sun
over endlessly blending shades of blues and whites, not caring
whether the day was beginning or ending. I liked exactly where

---

1 C.J. Jung, *Collected Works 7* (Princeton, New Jersey: Prince University
Press, 1966), 409.

I was, noticing the similarities between clouds billowing against the sky and snowy mountains rising up from the ocean. Being in such vast empty spaces of white fading into turquoise depths both above and below me, I felt suspended in time.

The pain in my back eventually forced me to move from my reverie and stagger down the aisle to the stewards' station, where my routine was to stretch and move for ten minutes every hour. The stewards explained that we were flying over Iceland into the sunrise, and would be landing a little before 9:00 A.M. in London. I felt thankful for my moment of time out of time, knowing that it would help me make the transition between such radically different worlds as the one I lived in and the one I was about to walk through. Until that moment over Iceland, I was still absorbed in my own familiar thoughts about all I had left behind with my family, friends, and clients. I could not yet fathom how I happened to be on this flight to London. Or why. In only a few hours we would be landing, and I would say good-bye to my traveling companion as she headed into London for her business meetings.

I had the sudden thought that I was to see beyond, or perhaps a larger picture than, the walking therapy that had been born from my back injury. Why else would I suddenly find myself being transported through time, space, and culture to walk side by side with strangers through England? Not as wounded healer attempting to heal myself and others, but as photojournalist who was to record with word and image whatever occurred on our journey together. Having a suspended moment gave me a chance to see and savor what was in the exact present, not what needed fixing, changing, or translating, but what was simply as it was. As the tour's photojournalist, I wanted to record what happened with as little interpretation as an imperfect human being can possibly have. I would do my best, all the while knowing that whatever I experienced would be filtered through plenty of my own personal biases and points of view. I wanted to feel fully in the moment as I had over Iceland, equanimous with all that was above and below, neither in past nor future time, and not longing for or regretting one thing or another.

By the time we landed in London, my walking companions would just be setting off from Cheltenham Spa for the first leg of a fifty-mile walk through the Cotswolds of England. We would be walking about ten miles per day for the next five days, but I would miss the first day's walk since I had another four hours' travel by bus, train, and taxi before I would arrive in Winchcombe. Continuing my journey, I noticed the country hillsides were like tapestries of bright yellow flowers, alternating with squares of green fields. Ancient stone walls divided properties filled with sheep, horses, or cows. In the villages, thatched roofs covered small stone houses along winding cobblestone streets. No superhighways to be seen, no shopping malls, bank machines, quick marts, or fast-food stores. In fact, the heart of England seemed to beat very slowly.

93

I felt my own body's rhythm match this beat easily, with gratitude. With no hurry, no push to get anywhere else or do anything other than be right here, *fast* had very suddenly and completely lost all significance. When I reached our meeting place near Sudley castle, I heard the meowing call of two white peacocks, eccentric guards patrolling the perimeters. I was greeted by one of the guides, who had spread a picnic out from the tailgate of her station wagon. Alice handed me a cup of barley water (lemonade) and a tin of biscuits (cookies) and said several other wayfarers had already arrived and were wandering about the castle. I could wait and meet each walker as he or she straggled in or I could go have a look at the castle—whatever suited me would be fine, she said. I felt eager to see how the first day's walk had been, so I stayed to meet everyone and hear the stories.

There were four men and ten women, from the ages of thirty-five to sixty-nine. Some experienced hikers and nature-lovers, while others had just completed their first daylong walk. They came from Australia, Austria, New Zealand, England, and America. Some were retired history and literary buffs; others were businessmen on vacation with their wives after meetings in London; a few were seasoned walking tour participants. There were Americans visiting Europe for the first time, singles on adventure with the hopes of meeting others, and there were people like me, wanting to heal an ailment or improve general health conditions. In the morning we all gathered after breakfast to check maps and hear plans for the day. We would be walking along the public path from Winchcombe to Stanway, where we would have our first rest stop for tea and biscuits, then on to Haille's Abbey, an ancient Cistercian Monastery.

As we headed down the cobblestone street toward the edge of town, where the public path joined with Pilgrim's Way, I realized with a surprise that my very first step on this week-long journey was that of the pilgrim's. No matter where I went, I did not seem to get very far away from the phenomenon of that word. I was beginning my walking tour with people from all over the world who had converged together to share vacation time as an outdoor adventure.

Our time together was not about focusing on healing, spirituality, psychotherapy, or the questing of a pilgrimage. Yet the sign marking our path clearly read, "Pilgrim's Way." Using my emerging philosophy of embracing all, I considered that every human was on a pilgrimage of sorts, no matter where we went, together or separately, whether we were well or sick, believers or disbelievers, rich or poor. Most of us, perhaps all of us, wanted to walk paths through life that allowed the fullest manifestation of the life force we could find, no matter what happened.

I paid attention to an evolving new language, beginning with the words *notitia* and "pilgrimage." Though I had no names yet for my developing philosophy of healing in relation to nature, I could say that the practice seemed pantheistic, from the Greek words *pan*, meaning "all," and *theistic*, meaning "god." Perhaps the reason I had no term to give to this new way of perceiving was that it had more to do with a sense of verb than noun, of noticing all that was alive in the present moment.

Embracing All

By practicing *notitia* of what was before us—seeing without preconceiving, whether in nature, in the office, or within ourselves—we would be able to sense at an instinctual level the wisdom inherent in a life force that moved all of us toward life. We humans were definitely connected to the stories of nature and vice versa, all of us part of a much larger whole, an immense interactional field. Certainly, we affected one another, whether or not our impact was metaphoric or actual. My own body's struggle to heal brought me time and again to the simple truth that to find my health again, I had to consider the whole, and how all parts related together in the present moment.

Learning Nature's Language

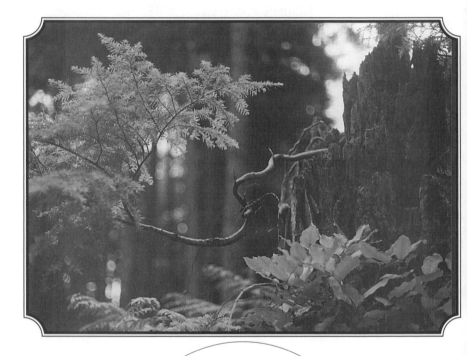

Nature's Language *appears to be
growing like a vine from its
nurse-log, when in fact the vine is the top of an invisible tree
growing from within the nurse-log,
with healthy branches visibly sprouting from the lower regions.*

Chapter 9

Upon returning home from my adventure in England, I felt a strong urge to redefine the language of psychotherapy so that it was more inclusive, less judgmental. I let nature show me how to use its lens for seeing into the present with as little preconception as possible. A spindly, young pine growing laterally from its slow-decaying, seven-foot-tall nurse-log gave me some clues on how to do this. I felt a bit sad that the vine-like tree might never turn and head upward in the direction of a free-standing tree. Because it had not developed its own base early on, it would likely continue reaching out like a branch to use the nurse-log as its permanent trunk. Though nurse-logs were very generous with themselves and their nutrients, providing a temporary foundation for new seedlings, there must be a turning point in the lives of all seedlings in which they find their own source from which to grow. Eventually, they must release the nurse-log, much like a child must wean from her mother. Not to do so created what I considered a parasitic life that might never become self-generative.

The little pine I watched stretching laterally probably had mistaken itself for a branch, not a tree. In human terms this would be called "confused identity." I thought this might be so partially because of the nurse-log's enormous size. The spindly little branch-tree was dwarfed by the mass under it, making it unlikely for its own roots to reach ground any time soon.

Or it might have been due to some early wound from inside the nurse-log that was not visible to me. The physics of gravity would eventually cause this little tree's reach to droop to the ground, forcing its branchlike trunk to grow downward in the opposite direction of a healthy tree, with no likely resolution other than a dysfunctional life, possibly a short one. But this would be using psychological language in describing nature. What I had been learning through my pilgrimage into nature was just the opposite of the preconceived judgments represented by clinical terms. Why not see what might happen if we interchanged nature's language with that of psychology? A fresh perspective seemed more possible when curiosity and discovery motivated understanding, rather than classification and diagnostics of the human condition.

For example, the branch-tree, with its impairment of identity, would be representative of what is termed for humans in psychiatric literature as a "a borderline personality." Such a pattern demonstrates a lack of identity and a desperate need to make use of other people's boundaries for a sense of self. A person who is thus motivated is likely to have missed out on consistent enough structure in his early life to find a solid foundation for growing into a sure sense of himself, of knowing where his own boundary lines end and another's begin. Understanding this makes relationships with people who struggle with the borderline phenomenon a far more compassionate process, especially since such dilemmas can be experienced as very difficult, unpredictable, and confusing to deal with.

Since such persons use others for their foundational support and self-identity when they are encouraged toward independence, they tend to feel this kind of support as a life-threatening abandonment from whomever they are bonded to. On the other hand, to collude by letting oneself be used for too long as a nurse-log prevents a borderline person from learning to thrive in his own right and learning to shape his own unique identity. This paradoxical dilemma often feels like a no-win, not only for the therapist and the client, but for all people who struggle with the borderline phenomenon, including friends and family members.

Reading the clues of people's current responses to life helps me understand what shaped them in the early years, which is useful not as an excuse for difficult or destructive behavior but as a compass guide for understanding the repetition motif. All of us, borderline or not, tend to repeat in our lives what we learned as children. This, of course, includes gift and wound. But the DSM-IV, a diagnostic manual for psychologists, describes pathology as if the borderline process were only a dysfunction, not a learned adaptation to a rather chaotic early life in which the child could not win for a number of different reasons. Such a child, later in life, tends to practice this no-win way of living like the branch-tree, until there is a radical intervention that forces a different turn toward life. Before that happens, borderline-type personalities often put their friends and family in plenty of losing situations in relation to them. They represent over and over again through current relationships what had happened to them as children, when there were few consistent clues about who was who and what was what. With such blurred identities, they often call forth the same difficult situations into the present as familiar, though chaotic, patterns.

99

When I have experienced myself as therapist, friend, or colleague in such a no-win, I finally recognize that somewhere in our dynamic there exists a borderline process. I see it as a verb, not a noun. The image of the lateral-reaching tree inspires me to ask myself, Where is the *choice-point* in this relationship where the boundary line between our two different lives has been blurred? Such a choice-point is often relational. The other person could not become too dependent unless I am too nurturing, and vice versa. Continuing to use nature's language, the lateral-growing tree, with its mistaken identity, is more likely to change its patterns when a portion of the nurse-log falls away, thus insisting that the life force of the pine mobilize on behalf of its own life. Without the foundation of another, the tree could not continue reaching laterally but would have to pull back to send life energy into creating a strong base for itself.

But abandonment is something that most of us try mightily to avoid either having done to us or doing to another, even when such an intervention might shock the life force into finding its right and healthy way. When I tend such phenomenon with the compass of the Hippocratic oath, *Above all else, do no harm,* I can usually find my way through working with the difficulties and confusions inherent in what's called the "borderline process." Paradoxically, it is sometimes more harmful to be helpful. Stepping away can occasionally force the painful process of another's having to distinguish the boundaries enough to find his own true identity. When the point of the therapeutic process is healing, I feel that our language needs to suggest how to turn on behalf of accessing the life force, of showing how we are all in this life together, and how we might help create each other through our interpersonal relationships.

In contrast, the following diagnostic language of the border-line disorder found in the *DSM-IV* describes such a person with borderline personality to be a solitary aberration, who is primarily dysfunctional and unaccountable.[1] This definition has given us no hints on how to relate to such a person with compassion and understanding:

1. frantic efforts to avoid real or imagined abandonment.
    Note: Do not include suicidal or self-mutilating
    behavior covered in criterion 5.
2. a pattern of unstable and intense interpersonal
    relationships characterized by alternating between
    extremes of idealization and devaluation
3. identity disturbance: markedly and persistently unstable
    self-image or sense of self

---

1 American Psychiatric Association, *Diagnostic and Statistical Manual of Mental Disorders*, 4th ed. (Washington, D.C.: American Psychological Association, 1994), 654.

4. impulsivity in at least two areas that are potentially self-damaging (e.g., spending, sex, substance abuse, reckless driving, binge eating) Note: Do not include suicidal or self-mutilating behavior covered in criterion 5
5. recurrent suicidal behavior, gestures, or threats, or self-mutilating behavior
6. affective instability due to a marked reactivity of mood (e.g., intense episodic dysphoria, irritability, or anxiety usually lasting a few hours and only rarely more than a few days)
7. chronic feelings of emptiness
8. inappropriate, intense anger or difficulty controlling anger (e.g., frequent displays of temper, constant anger, recurrent physical fights)
9. transient, stress-related paranoid ideation or severe dissociative symptoms

Such a language system does not offer much insight into healing, which makes me wonder if its purpose is not more for the tension relief of an upset therapist than for the upset client. When I have tried to treat clients from within this language frame, the therapy fails in time. Many colleagues have suggested that this is so because the prognosis for change is not very high with the borderline pattern of dysfunction. Though this may be true, I also know that when I work with this phenomenon successfully, it is usually because I am willing to read the client's responses to life as if they were like trees walking. I am curious and compassionate, not reactive or judgmental, though most certainly their patterns can be alternately baffling, frightening, and just plain irritating when I hold an idea of how they are *supposed* to behave, and then do not. When I am able to recognize that certain responses they have to life represent what is happening within them, I feel far more compassionate than annoyed.

Using nature's language, I might rewrite the *DSM-IV* diagnostic criteria in a new way. Instead of describing chronic feelings of emptiness and boredom, I might say,

> With the borderline struggle, a person is showing us
> how it felt to him as a child to have no one certain
> to count on, no place to go for soothing. He has not
> yet learned how to calm himself when alone. His
> parent was too chaotic or absent for bonding to be
> a safe endeavor. He simply waited in emptiness to see
> what might happen, what might come forth from the
> other, not the self.

Or another rewrite from the perspective of symptom as symbol
might go like this:

> An early sense of abandonment made this person par-
> ticularly reactive and avoidant of re-experiencing such
> a threat, perceived or imagined, to his basic survival.

102   When I have been able to walk with such persons along
these difficult borders, reading their responses as signs along
the way, I am often able to see what kind of new life wants
to express itself beyond repetitive patterns. This is only true if
I \am not trying to encircle them within the boundary of the
psychiatric language system, though. If we in the profession of
psychology are able to access the client's creative imperative,
success often follows.

And we must be willing for this to happen imperfectly, as in
the case of Jonathan, who suffered the early loss of his father.
Jonathan's father had died shortly after Jonathan was born,
which put his mother into a crisis that completely destabilized
not only his early years but much of his childhood, up until he
was nine years old, when she remarried. With no other financial
support until then, Jonathan's mother had to work full time,
which meant that in some ways he lost both mother and father
in his formative years. By the time his mother had remarried,
Jonathan had already learned to make use of any situation that
presented itself for the caretaking of his needs. In fact, he became
obsessed with being taken care of by another. This pattern

became the shape of his life, seeking always to merge with another, panicking when too alone, cycling through one relationship after another until the age of forty-five, when his live-in lover, Linda, asked him to go to therapy with her. He had not sought it on his own because his identity was more directed toward others than toward self. She forced the issue, and he cooperated by participating with her in couples therapy.

Her complaints had to do with the amount of alcohol he consumed and his erratic mood swings, which seemed unrelated to anything that was going on in their life together. He admitted that he tried to control his drinking by not doing it in front of her. But when she found empty bottles of liquor around the house and was dismayed by the amount of time he needed to get going in the morning, she concluded that alcohol was a real problem. Jonathan could not see it as a problem since it had not yet become one to him. He hoped Linda would just calm down about it. His lack of insight was astounding to her, especially since he had seemed so sensitive at the beginning of the relationship. I asked when things had begun to change for her and was not surprised to hear that it was almost immediately after he moved into her house and began sitting around, whittling wood while watching television. Once he had found his nurse-log, he seemed to have lost the urge to impress her with his sensitivity and intelligence, which was in fact one of his many undeveloped gifts.

After hearing the history of Jonathan's relationships, I realized that he fit five of the diagnostic criteria of a borderline personality disorder, but this did not help Jonathan and Linda, who had come to me for therapy. What helped them most was for her to stop trying to take care of him. When she was finally able to do so, he found another woman to live with, and Jonathan's sad pattern persisted for another round. In paying attention to what was happening on the borderlines of Jonathan's life, I recognized in the process of his coming together, then apart, with Linda, that for a short while he had reclaimed woodcarving, something he had loved to do as a child. This interest over the years had gradually developed in Jonathan a real talent as a woodcarver. Even with little passion for it, he still created the most exquisite abstract shapes.

Using nature's language in describing this man's struggle, I'll say his life seemed to be parallel to the branch-tree's. If some part of his caretaking system were to fall away, he might be forced to access enough of his own life force to save himself. His relationship fell away, but his alcohol use and need to find another caretaker persisted, unfortunately. Before he terminated his therapy, I recommended that he quit drinking alcohol altogether with the support of AA, and that he pursue woodcarving with a mentor. Since Jonathan never called again, I do not know what happened next in his life, but I feel hopeful for him every time I walk by the little branch-tree.

I realized recently that this kind of thinking must be a form of prayer. I considered him with such unfounded hope, not for a change in his life patterns so much as for him to let his one generative urge thrive. I was so surprised to recognize how my worry had transformed to prayer with the inspiration of nature's language. The next time I passed by the branch-tree, I noticed a strong pine branch about three feet up from the ground insisting its way through the trunk of the nurse-log. *Aha*, I said to myself—perhaps Jonathan's growth was internal and invisible to us, and we would one day see who had been developing all along in spite of all odds, within the protection of the nurse-log that would one day fall away organically and in its own time.

Sheryl's struggle involved a different kind of borderline process than Jonathan's, though she, too, met five out of the eight criteria for such a diagnosis in the psychology manual. Her story was more like a cedar tree that had attached to a nurse-log early in its life but was eventually able to become free standing on its own. Without becoming fully merged, the seedling could draw out the nutrients from the nurse-log, thus preserving an identity to carry its life force upward. Sheryl came to see me for therapy at the height of her despair over being left by the man she hoped to marry. They had been together for several years and were engaged to be married, but her fiancé wanted to be sure before making a commitment. For him this meant dating another woman before settling down. Sheryl decided to wait, in the hopes that he would see the light sooner rather than later. Six

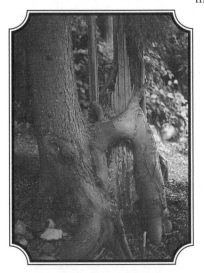

months later, he still had not decided, which was when Sheryl sought therapy for herself, concerned about her insomnia, rage explosions, weight loss, and substance use to numb what had become now-constant pain and anxiety.

When I learned to read Sheryl's responses as clues to the inner life or early sense of wound, her behavior patterns made very clear sense. She was demonstrating over and over again what it had felt like to her as a child to have suddenly lost the only world she knew when her mother abandoned the family. For several years following,

105

Attachment *made use of the nourishment from its nurse-log while establishing its own roots, creating an interesting sculpture at a co-housing community, composed of eight homes clustered around a shared common area. Langley, Washington.*

Sheryl and her father had lived in a state of chaos. Though he eventually remarried and the new stepfamily stabilized to become a strong support for everyone, those few years from age two to five were wounding to Sheryl. Fortunately, the first two years of life that preceded Sheryl's wounding allowed her enough stability and sense of identity to find her way in life. This was only shaken when the early loss was restimulated by the current loss of her fiancé.

She was able to make use of therapy to help stabilize herself, just as the cedar had done with the nurse-log.

Until Sheryl met another man, whom she eventually married, her erratic patterns were extremely difficult to work with in therapy. I had not yet learned at the time that the no-win with a borderline process simply demonstrated the inner conflict turned outside, so we could see and understand with more compassion. When I could read her responses in this way, I felt far more loving, less judgmental, and more fully able to be present with her process. I finally realized that success in her mind was not a satisfactory completion of a therapeutic process, as it had been in mine. Her goal was to find another relationship. When she did find one and could finally release the old one, she abruptly left therapy. This left me reverberating in shock until I understood that she was showing by her behavior what had happened to her as a young child, having been left so abruptly and permanently. I could respond with more compassion to these difficult situations by using nature's language to understand and make meaning of them.

New Life in Relationships

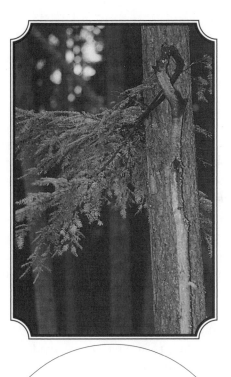

Creative Relationship *struggles to grow*

in the shade of another tree.

To thrive,

it made a loop with its topmost branch to stretch laterally into its

own sunlight.

Langley, Washington.

Chapter 10

Though most libraries and bookstores housed huge sections of self-help books focusing on how to have, improve, save, and leave intimate relationships, I had yet to find any wiser advice than the stories I stumbled across in nature. Trees lived creatively from the very particular places from which they grew, no matter what was happening around them. Rarely did I see relationships between trees to be perfect or even close to ideal. Such a concept was absent in nature because the trees were simply striving toward the real. They did so in imperfectly beautiful ways, like the young pine that made a looping turn at the very top of its life in order to grow laterally into the light. This young pine had found itself struggling to survive in the shadow of its massive elder. To continue growing along the genetically programmed pathway straight upward would have meant certain death. For this tree to live within a relationship, it had to become extremely creative. It turned a somersault into the sunlight available. I marveled at the genius of such a creative solution.

One of my clients was finally able to discover a miraculous turn in her life when, as a single parent, she adopted a child from China. For years she tried in vain to find a relationship with a man and have a family, but time had ticked right past her child-bearing years. Though she had many interesting relationships with lovers, none had become marriage partners. She did not want this fact to interfere with her deepest heart's desire to be a mother, so she turned directly toward her dream and adopted a child. Within two years of the extraordinary challenges of being a single mother, she met a man who wanted to share family life with her. It was her radical turn toward new life which had brought her to what she could not find by walking the more traditional path. Such a turn revealed her genius, though at times, I am sure she would say that being a single mother also revealed her biggest flaws.

A couple I worked with for several years had come together just after losing their long-term partners for very different reasons. Instead of proceeding down the traditional path of falling in love and marrying, these two decided they wanted to let their relationship tell them what form it wanted, very much like a poet lets a poem reveal its native form. For the second half of their lives, they decided to maintain separate homes and spend time together that had nothing to do with problem-solving different parenting styles or financial strategies, or psychological issues that manifested themselves in their intimacy. Both decided to do their personal work with their own therapists, and see what it was like to experience intimacy as more pleasure than problem and conflict.

This did not mean they avoided difficult times; rather, that they handled them differently than they had in their previous marriages, often asking the gods for help in the midst of a conflict. Rather than scapegoating each other when threatened and fighting from opposite positions, they prayed together and were silent. Then they might dance or go kayaking, or walking, or share their dreams or make love. In any case, they made a point not to follow old patterns of projecting themselves or their shadows onto the other. What emerged from this relationship was a nurturance of one another's spirituality and generativity, which gave them both time and space to tend to their artistic interests.

Not every couple I worked with had such freedom of choice. As with trees in the forest, people found themselves in relationships that were far from ideal; but unlike trees, people could get

109

up and leave relationships that were too troublesome. I pondered such a scenario at Carkeek Park one day with a friend who had come with me to share a picnic lunch and watch the salmon spawn. She was contemplating the ending of a relationship. It was September and the air was warm and clean. The leaves on the trees had not yet changed into their fall colors, but the salmon had already begun to swim upstream. Our conversation drifted back and forth between our surroundings in the present and the different dramas of our lives. I gave her an update on the healing of my back and told her about how restored I had felt standing next to the tree near my house following the trauma of my MRI. The forty-year-old weeping willow had not only helped me but provided housing for an extended family of raccoons who looked like benign little bandits draped in the upper branches. I marveled at how willows could create such a great canopy of leaves descending into almost perfect symmetry, like gigantic umbrellas.

My friend, who was about to leave her partner, clearly did not feel as magnanimous as I felt that day.

She shrugged, "Not always." Gesturing to the weeping willow next to our picnic table, she said, "Case in point."

The willow was not symmetrical at all. We both got up to investigate. Standing next to its trunk and staring up into its overhead branches, we could see a snarled tangle rising upward, not downward. Something had stimulated this tree to do the opposite of creating a descending canopy of leaves, at least on one side of it. Stepping away from the trunk, I could see that an alder that was growing along the stream, about thirty feet away, had leaned into the willow's light. Its upper branches rested on the willow, blocking about a third of its sunlight. The lack of symmetry was explained.

My friend was immediately judgmental and annoyed with the alder for interfering with the willow's life. I knew she felt this way about her partner, who had dominated their relationship. "The parks department should remove that alder," she said.

110

But I wanted to spend some time imagining how the natural course of life might handle this dilemma without intervention from an outside force, such as a chain saw. My friend wandered upstream to watch the salmon spawn while I stayed to read the story of this relationship of trees. Still amazed at her annoyance with the poor old leaning alder, I walked over to examine its base. Perhaps it was already dying, and should be taken down so the willow could thrive. But if this were not a city park constantly tended, replanted, and pruned, how would nature solve this seemingly disastrous relationship? The alder was living close to the stream and seemed healthy with plenty of water close to its roots. But the soil was so damp it had not been sturdy enough to hold the height of such a fast-growing alder. Had it not been for the willow, the alder probably would have fallen hard to the ground. Growing at an angle, it would do fine for years to come.

What about the willow? Surely it was destined to live a life beyond supporting the life of another. Strolling back to the willow, I contemplated the underside of its umbrella for a long time before I understood the genius in this relationship between two trees. Where the alder rested, the willow had twisted, reversing its branches to grow upward, extending itself higher than the point of their meeting. That was not just a snarl of tangled branches as I had first thought. It was how the willow created a most original solution that honored the lives of two, not just one. By stretching taller it would eventually be able to drape a cascading canopy of leaves down over the alder, thus making an even larger symmetry than it was born to do. The alder had made this challenge possible, and the willow simply incorporated it all into life. They had come together to thrive, turning wound to gift, making use of their innermost resources.

They inspired me to look at human relations differently. I wondered how my friend might see what was being challenged in herself to grow enough to meet her seemingly over-dominant partner. If she could open up possibilities beyond her defensive judgments, what might happen? What genius might be born?

I knew it was not yet time to have such a discussion with my friend, so I mused instead about a couple I had worked with several years before. George, a middle-aged, semiretired businessman who no longer needed to work, wanted a meaningful relationship most in his life. He hoped he had found this with Steve, who was fifteen years younger and at the height of his career in dentistry.

They had very different lifestyles, which made them uncertain about proceeding with a partnership. George wanted to travel and enjoy his hard-earned leisure time with a mate who also wanted to explore life beyond work. Steve loved to travel and wanted to share life with George, but he still had massive debts to pay off from his education and specialty training. He could not put the number of hours into dentistry to pay off loans quickly because of recurring headaches from a collapsed cervical disc in his spine. Leaning forward to look into patients' mouths for hours on end had become an occupational hazard for Steve, who alternated between working hard to keep up financially, then falling behind when his physical disability took him over with excruciating pain.

Both George and Steve had vulnerabilities they did not want the other to see. When they came to me for psychotherapy, both were frightened about revealing themselves. George worried about being considered an insignificant old man, no longer in the fast lane of a very competitive business, and Steve worried about being a failure at the business he had put so much into developing. It seemed clear to me they had come together in hopes of turning their vulnerabilities into gift, not curse. But they did not know how to do anything but fight against what they considered to be weaknesses or flaws in themselves that they did not want the other to see. Fortunately, over time, they were able to risk having a look at vulnerability as part of a meaningful relationship. When they did, it proved to be the new life waiting to blossom.

By new life, I meant the accessing of the resources that brought forth what was most original in each of them. Their creative solution, similar to the willow and the alder, had to do with George's accepting his retirement, resting into trusting his relationship with Steve enough to be fully himself. He encouraged Steve to do the same, which was a bit more of a struggle, just as it was for the willow. Steve could not settle for just abandoning his career and letting George take care of finances, though there was more than plenty to go around. Instead, he sold his business, paid off his debts, and shared the finances with George while going back to school. Following a lifelong dream of being an actor, he chose drama school and challenged himself to grow in ways he had never thought possible. Their convergence at midlife, though certainly not perfect or problem-free, emerged as great gift for both, but only because they could recognize and love what the other originally thought of in himself as flaw. Their relationship helped them honor such vulnerability as the doorway into what was most original in both.

Not many couples consider marrying their partners' shadows. Usually, we choose the sun side in relationship and are surprised to find shade in our partners or ourselves. But sometimes, as with nature, such a discovery can bring about a better balance in relationship. One particular couple had been married for twelve years and had shared the running of a cottage-style industry from their home. Suddenly, they faced bankruptcy following the husband's almost-fatal car accident. Martha had to spend her time tending to her husband Bill, who had previously been the primary mover and shaker of their business. He was the more extroverted of the two and by far the more courageous risk taker in the world of work.

But over the months of his recuperation, they both discovered that he had lost his confidence and could not concentrate on even the familiar mundane tasks of accounting for the business. Martha panicked at first, but soon had to get on with life. If she did not, they both would not make it. Bill now depended on her. While he stayed at home and tried to get well, Martha closed their business down and went to work for a temporary agency. This meant Bill had to find something to do with himself alone at home that had nothing to do with work. Both were extremely uncomfortable with this role reversal for a number of reasons, but there were no other options for them. They had to look within their own undeveloped sides, their shadows, to find something new they could rely on.

Bill found a musician-poet within himself that never would have emerged had he continued in business, and Martha probably would not have found the part of herself that could thrive well in her own right. She had depended so much on Bill's extroverted energy that she had not developed her own confidence in running things. Her first employer at the temp agency recognized her quiet, calm, and very efficient skills in management and hired her full-time to run the office. Not every couple could rise to meet this kind of challenge. Often, what happened with such radical reversals was a split-up of the marriage. For something creative to emerge within relationship required both partners to uncover a mysterious and original force within that would benefit both. Usually, this would be a surprise to each, not anything they would have planned for or even wanted beforehand, but something they were able to manifest in a shared creative process.

A friend of mine once put a hilarious personal ad in a weekly that read, "Full-bodied woman, not necessarily athletic, with a great sense of humor, looking for same in man." That was all. She figured such an ad would rule out anyone but the exact man she wanted to meet, one who was not looking for perfection or an ideal relationship. She wanted to introduce the parts of herself, first, that more likely lived in the shadows or were not all that acceptable. For her this was about not being the size and shape of a model. It was about being real, talents and flaws included. Inviting vulnerability into relationship from the start made it possible for her to meet someone who shared her value of authenticity over perfection. She married the first man who answered her ad, and together they have created a generous extended family that celebrates what is most original in each, no matter how eccentric, genius-like, or ordinary that might be. Like a healthy cedar grove, their family keeps growing.

CHAPTER 11
Coming Apart, Lush with Life

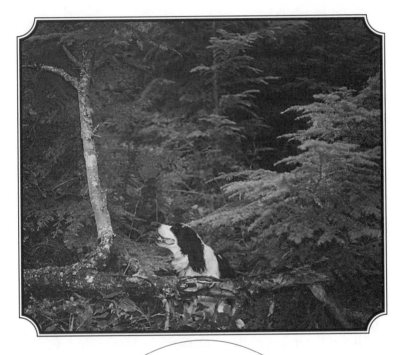

Falling into New Life

found a way to thrive beyond its destruction

by staying partially rooted.

Having been pushed to the ground with its topmost branches twisted

and broken off, this tree transformed its remaining

two branches into thriving trunks.

Langley, Washington.

Chapter 11

Marilyn and Greg's marriage was like a tree leaning precipitously on the side of a hill. It did not take much for it to topple over completely. I wanted to try using my nature lens for viewing the coming apart of their relationship from a perspective other than taking sides, making judgments, giving advice, even trying to save them from themselves. More essentially, I wanted to see what might follow naturally, since divorce seemed to be destiny for both of them for different reasons. Their divorce reminded me of a young twenty-year-old pine which had fallen or been pushed over and was lying parallel to the ground. From its horizontal trunk, two branches had turned to grow straight upward. The top of the tree must have once stretched across the trail, but someone had broken and twisted it back to die. Miraculously, this tree continued to thrive with no base and no top. The remaining fifteen feet of its trunk supported the lives of two branches whose cells had transformed into trunk cells. One of those branch-trees stood eight feet tall, and the other about four feet tall, both lush with life. This is exactly what followed several years after Marilyn and Greg's divorce.

Two years before their split, Greg's mother had died at about the time his third daughter was born by Caesarean section. While immersed in the shock and grief of his mother's death, he also had to tend to his recovering wife, their newborn, a two-year-old toddler, and a five-year-old. Though devastated by grief, he blocked out all else but caretaking, as if he had become mother himself. Because his wife could not lift any of the children while she healed from surgery, Greg took an indefinite sabbatical from his work to be nursemaid for the whole family. He would bathe and dress the newborn, then deliver her to his wife for nursing, all the while making sure the toddler stayed out of mischief and the five-year-old had a ride to kindergarten. Instead of bemoaning his fate, Greg, thrilled to discover how much he loved being at home with the children, said he wished his wife would go back to work one day and let him stay home to be Mr. Mom. This happened, but it came through another unexpected tragedy, not a wish come true.

With no warning, Marilyn moved out of the house one day with all the children and most of the furniture. Beyond devastated with this second loss, Greg, who had for years refused to do couples counseling with Marilyn, now proposed family therapy, promising to do whatever would bring his family back together. They did this for six months while living in separate homes and sharing custody of the children, but reconciliation did not occur. Friends and family alike were sad for them, as they were for themselves at first. But over time they both realized they had come together mainly to be parents, not intimate partners. They were incompatible as husband and wife, but unusually good friends as parents. By drawing on the extended families for support, Marilyn was able to go back to work and Greg could continue to be both mother and father to his children at least 50 percent of the time.

For several years, the difficulties in Greg's life looked like the fallen tree with its top wrenched and broken back, but when we looked closely enough, we could see where creativity emerged in the whole family. Though he valued the nuclear family as a concept, Greg recognized that had he and Marilyn stayed together, their children would not be thriving as well as they were with the generosity and interest of both extended families. Both sets of grandparents not only felt themselves to be suddenly wanted and needed; they were essential in the lives of the broken family. By meeting this challenge the grandparents had become truly generative in their senior years, becoming more energetic as a result. Greg and Marilyn, who honored their children's needs first, made a point of sharing holidays, birthdays, and school events together, not insisting on the tug-of-war which is typical of many who refuse reunion long after a divorce. Greg and Marilyn abided by what was most original in themselves, not by the status quo of divorces. Their wholeheartedness made it possible for all to thrive, especially the children who felt loved fully by both sides of the family.

When Marilyn began working for an airline, she made certain that all benefits covered Greg, too, so he and the children could enjoy vacations together. Greg was always generous about including Marilyn in the videos he filmed of the children's special events. Both were consistently more concerned about collaborating successfully on raising their children than they were about sustaining old patterns or wounds from their now defunct marriage. Thus, their divorce made it possible to be far more creative together raising children. Though neither was living the life they had imagined, they could celebrate without reservation the richness of the treasures they did share. Two unusual trees lush with life.

Not many relationships could be counted on for staying together, nor should they, as was true for Greg and Marilyn. Some couples simply could not thrive with one another no matter what changes they tried to make together or separately. Though divorce was almost always difficult to go through, it could also become the way for some couples to find the genius of their relationship. This seemed more likely to happen when both persons were willing to look within themselves for the life force essential for growing in another direction, and were also willing to share what they found with the beloved other, as was true for Marilyn and Greg.

The exception to this would be when one or both of the ex-partners were unable to experience empathy for the other. Then what might be engendered instead would be a holocaust of hatred and annihilation of anything that might be ready for birth between them, devastating the regeneration of both lives. Even without empathy, though, if the partners were still willing to share a process that honored the time it took to separate one's roots and make the transplanting safe for both parties, then devastation could be avoided. This often requires the extra support or mediation of psychotherapy to assure that one person's life is not simply sacrificed to save the other's, as in war. Nature's lens can be very helpful in perceiving another way to separate lives. The couples I have known who were most successful at coming apart intact have followed the basic principles of transplanting. They carefully consider timing, making certain the plant is dormant so its roots do not go into shock because of a too-rapid change of climate.

Frank and Denise, who met each other as seniors in high school, decided to go to the same college and share a room together. They found each other to be so compatible that their close friendship very quickly evolved into intimacy. After a year they made a commitment to monogamy, and both imagined marriage at some point in the future, but they never actually got around to taking that extra step. Thirteen years of sharing their lives in a basically contented relationship brought them into psychotherapy to choose between three options as presented by Denise: Get married and start a family, proceed as they were, or separate to explore other options. Frank felt paralyzed by having to decide when he was not clear about any of the three possibilities. Their relationship up to this point in time had helped them both grow into successful adulthoods, but it also had been what is called in psychological terms a merged relationship. Denise was ready to step into new territory, but Frank was afraid to do anything different, to make any decisions that might take them out of the easy flow of life he felt with Denise. I recommended that they both do individual therapy, if they could, while I met with them as a couple once a month for a year.

During that time, it became clear that they needed to know themselves better before they could take any steps toward changing their relationship. They decided to try living separately for six months to a year, continue with their commitment to one another, and see if the space helped them differentiate enough to make some decisions. They helped each other move into their separate homes. Kindness and consideration was primary to them as a couple, to such a degree that they were willing to defer their own needs for the other's, which made decision-making so difficult. Having separate living spaces gave them a chance to focus more on themselves for a change. In some ways, this couple was so intertwined they needed a bit of pruning in order to grow further. They did so tenderly and over a long time period, so that each felt supported and loved as they let go of some old patterns that were familiar but no longer life-enhancing to them.

Eventually they discovered they were on different life paths altogether but still loved one another. Frank wanted to travel and experiment with other ways of living his life. In particular, he wanted to explore another career that might take him out of the country for extended time periods. Denise had come to the conclusion that she was ready for a family and did not want to wait any longer. Both were still young enough to pursue their different dreams and start over with another partner. They set each other free without causing harm, as so often happens when the process is not a shared one.

With Sally and Chris, a couple who had been together for almost fifteen years, something similar happened, but not so consciously as with Frank and Denise. Chris had been recruited by her company to take a promotion that meant moving to another city. She and Sally faced the choice of moving together or separating temporarily to decide how to proceed after a year. They separated, though this was quite traumatic for Sally. A year later, when they faced the choice about how to proceed with a long-distance relationship, Sally decided she could no longer be in such a partnership. They had serious heartbreak to contend with. Having barely survived the first shocking transplant of their relationship, of separating their interlinking root system, Sally knew that to survive, she must stay in one place and let her own roots sink deeply into the ground as a solitary tree. Both women still loved one another and made certain over the next few years that the other was supported through the changes in their relationship, no matter how differently each needed to live. Empathy was part of their relationship as lovers and in the transition to friendship as well. Above all, they took all the time they needed to process this significant transition in both of their lives. The transplanting thrived.

Sometimes, what draws a couple together is the very thing that also brings them apart at another stage in life. Two artists, Connie and Tom, who met and married just after graduating with MFA degrees in visual art, helped each other develop their artistic careers. But when it came to the daily grind of living together and making a living, they found themselves competing at almost every turn. By the time they were both successfully established with their art careers, they had lost interest in one another intimately. Yet neither wanted to lose the other as a beloved friend with whom they had walked through such a significant time in their lives. They committed to a year of psychotherapy to help decide how to proceed in a way that would be supportive of one another and the lives they had created. Their counselor helped them tend to old habits and patterns differently enough that by the end of the year they were able to draw up divorce papers with no battle at all. The genius of this relationship was birthed in its ending, as they finally learned how to accept and truly respect their differences.

There is a wisdom in making the endings of relationships as sacred as the beginnings; of being certain that transplanting takes as much time and careful tending as an original planting might take; of not making judgments about relationships coming apart or staying together, but simply watching what follows to see the innate wisdom of each story.

CHAPTER 12
Voice of the Vulnerable

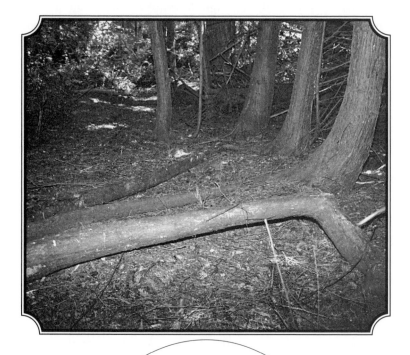

Source Tree *grows from*
an invisible source buried deep underground.
Four root-like trunks run
from this point along the ground for about ten feet before they
turn to grow upright, creating an abundant cedar grove.
Hedgebrook Cottages, Langley, Washington.

Chapter 12

When I was granted a month-long writing residency at Hedgebrook Cottages on Whidbey Island, I started each writing day by taking my morning cup of coffee with me to sit amidst the roots of a cedar grove. My back had healed enough for me to sit fairly comfortably for longer than an hour at a time. After contemplating my surroundings, I would close my eyes and listen more deeply within, then begin to write about the interweaving life stories of people and the natural world. The cedar grove itself became one of those stories. When I had first come across it during a walk in the woods, I had no idea it was a grove at all. It looked like a clearing in the forest with three twenty-foot logs angling out from a center point on the ground. Though their symmetry seemed measured, I noticed on second glance that the logs had not been arranged by human hand. They were live, gigantic roots emerging from an unknown source below the ground.

For a moment I imagined an upside-down story where trees grew from within the earth and their roots broke through into the outer world to reveal what usually could not be perceived. Curious about these roots that seemed to have a life of their own, I followed one along its path to an endpoint twenty feet away, where it turned radically at a ninety-degree angle to became a cedar tree standing over thirty feet tall. From the base of this tree, another root extended itself three feet to the left, providing enough space for yet another cedar tree to thrive at its side. Tracing the paths of each main root to its endpoint, I found similar, but unique, stories of life. The immense root on the right made a lovely, aesthetic flourish with a rising arch before descending into the ground to provide nourishment for the twin trunks to which it had given birth. The middle root did what many siblings do who find themselves between two others. They balanced, or filled in, what needed completion to make the family whole. What grew from the endpoint of the middle root besides the tallest cedar tree was an addendum-root, extending along the ground to its left, from which grew another thirty-foot-tall cedar. Thus, three roots emerging from an invisible source underground had given birth to a grove of seven trees. These in turn sculpted all their trunks and branches together in a communal effort to create the shape of one large tree. Each had extended a piece of itself to bring forward new life, just as the original tree had done for them.

124

I felt certain that, long ago, an immense and majestic old-growth cedar had been standing where I stood, at the source point of the giant roots. Because the forest had been replanted and cleared several times since her day, there was no longer any sign of even a stump to show where she might have been—only the remnants of a root system that continued to live underground until it was time for new life to emerge. Miraculous. I was on sacred ground. Asking the life force that mysteriously thrived underground, on earth, and in the skies to be present while I wrote, I returned every morning to the "source tree" with my cup of coffee, yellow legal pad, and pens to record the emerging stories. Though I did not know how it might be manifest at the time, I felt that the cedar grove, with its interconnecting roots and branches, was revealing how we were linked, inspired, nourished, and sheltered by one another in community.

Whenever I spent time writing from this source tree, I found that what wanted to be voiced would come from a deeper place within myself, not always about the trees or my clients or my own healing journey. Sometimes, I recognized a connection between what was very personal and what might also be universal. After one of my morning meditations by the cedar, I walked down to the farmhouse to make a phone call and passed by the goat yard. I noticed that the goats were still locked inside their shed, knocking from inside. I wanted to release them but hesitated, not wanting to interfere with the farm's routine. In just that moment, like a hot poker sizzling, an unbearably painful childhood memory burst through to singe my heart. I could almost not tolerate the internal pain, true and fresh as if it had happened in that moment.

My sister, age eight, and I, age six, had adopted a six-week-old kitten, fluffy, gray, striped. My sister and I were sleeping together in our parents' bed that night, which meant they may have been away while we had an overnight babysitter. We had put the kitten to sleep in a wicker laundry basket in the bathroom with soft cloths and a little ticking clock to remind him of his mother's heartbeat. He meowed, but we had been told to let him cry until he went to sleep, or else he would learn to wake us up every night. The person from whom we had adopted the kitten said it was natural for a baby to cry during his first night away from his mother. But soon the kitten would be comfortable in his new home, and we could feed and play with him in the morning.

Meow, meow. I lay stiffly in bed trying not to listen, but hearing every pitiful little mew. I forced myself to stay in bed, fighting against the hard tug toward the kitten. I whispered reassurances from the bedroom that he was not alone, that we would feed him first thing in the morning. Meow, meow. Every cell in my body stood on alert, unable to relax until the kitten fell asleep.

After what seemed like days to me, I heard silence. When the sun finally rose, I was first out of bed and into the bathroom to greet the kitten. He was not in his basket. I called for him, but lost my breath instead. His little body floated in the toilet. I picked him up, rubbed frantically with a towel, but it was far too late to save him. If I had responded when he first cried for help, I would not be holding his soggy, lifeless body, eyes glazed, tiny mouth open, spilling water from a swollen belly. My sobs awoke my sister, who staggered in and huddled with me over the dead kitten.

We took turns holding him, drying his fur, telling him how sorry we were. We said, *We didn't know you were crying for help. We would have come right away if we'd known you'd fallen in the toilet. We should have come, anyway. Oh, kitty, why did you climb out of your basket? We thought you were too little to crawl up the sides. We should not have had the basket so close to the toilet. Why didn't we let you sleep with us?*

The endless whys we asked each other that day forced us to accept every agonizing detail of the part we played in this tragedy. Our tears, which came and went throughout the week, did nothing to relieve my inner torture over this kitten's death. We gave him a special funeral and burial, but the hurt in my heart had never gone away, even remembering it almost forty years later. Such a wound was permanent, I thought. The image of that little gray, striped, kitten, sopping wet, struggling in vain to crawl up the slick sides of the toilet, mewing pitifully for his life, was indelible in my heart. When the hot poker of memory seared into me, I asked to be shown whatever I must learn and not forget in the kitten's memory.

What I heard from deep within was: *Always respond to the voice of the vulnerable.*

Reflecting back on my life, I realized that every significant turn I made had been shaped by this message, whether it had been in taking care of my animals, leaving a campsite, or deciding on a psychotherapy career. My writing had been a way to voice the vulnerable as well, not only in myself but often on behalf of those who had no voice. The kitten's message from so many years ago continued to shape my life, but that day at Hedgebrook it broke through as a direct command for the first time, *Always respond to the voice of the vulnerable.* I hoped my writing would be just such a response, whether this meant the vulnerable in human, plant, or animal.

I wanted to redefine the word, since the dictionary described "vulnerable" in the negative only, suggesting to me that our culture perceived vulnerable as "not valuable": "susceptible to physical injury, attack. Liable to succumb to censure or criticism. Assailable," (from the American Heritage Dictionary, Second College Edition). What if the definition were turned around so that the attackee, the vulnerable, were seen as more powerful, to be responded to first? My definition of vulnerable in the positive would be: *Natural, soul-like, exposed, open, not hidden, without armor, available, not to be assailed.* I had learned at age six, under the unknowingly destructive power of my sister's and my rules of management, of going against our instincts, of not responding to the call of the vulnerable, that life cannot be called back.

When I read this story along with several others about the interaction between humans and nature to an audience at Eliot Bay Book Company in Seattle, I received a flood of mail. Every response included a personal story about being vulnerable with nature. Some even sent photographs of their special trees with descriptions that revealed profound and affectionate bonds with the natural world. They were people who had discovered nature's generous offerings and wanted to share what they had noticed, reflecting a real desire for passing along the gifts they too had discovered. Their responses reminded me of the source tree, where I had wondered how we were all interconnected, even when we could not see the source that connected us.

I returned from my writing residency with a renewed devotion to trusting and listening to the voice of the vulnerable as a threshold into originality, as a source-point, as a gift of life to hear, see, and more essentially to respond to with love. My challenge was to bridge this truth for my clients, many of whom sought therapy for relief of what they considered to be intolerable vulnerability. Though David first came to psychotherapy in hopes of preparing himself to be an adoptive parent at midlife, our work together was about learning to love the vulnerable in ourselves. Unbeknownst to both of us, we stepped into a crucible of healing over the next few years which paralleled the stages of transformation I had witnessed in trees creating new life in response to their wounds. We learned to listen closely to the voice of the vulnerable within and were guided directly to the source of his creativity.

Unable to conceive a child of their own, David and his partner of twelve years had spent the past ten years pursuing adoption. Both were teachers and had the generosity of spirit, down-to-earth parenting skills, and stability of lifestyle that would have made them good parents. But they were considered by adoption agencies as *too old* at fifty. They had tried being foster parents for awhile, but found the lack of permanence far too difficult, the inevitable good-byes excruciating after opening their hearts so fully to children who came to stay only for awhile. Over the years, opportunities for private adoptions had almost became manifest, but for one reason or another, they collapsed at the last minute. This repeating, seemingly endless, cycle of hope, disappointment, then hope again, had occurred too many times, and David finally fell into despair himself. When he finally let go of his lifelong dream of having a child, he plummeted.

Though I did not share this with David, I too, had given up on conceiving a child of my own. But I had been blessed to share the parenting of my partner's five children. My personal loss remained significant to me, though, and probably would always be so. What wisdom could I share with David about what still grieved me so profoundly? Before I accepted David into therapy I consulted my supervising analyst, thinking it might be best to refer David to another therapist, one who was not also grieving her own loss. But he urged me to consider that because of our similar struggle, I might be more, rather than less, able to walk with a transforming kind of empathy down this path with him. Such is the way of the wounded healer. What happened in working with David over the next three years went far beyond the motif of wounded healer. We shared what I considered to be a sacred collaboration, peering together into nature for guidance.

When David and his partner emptied and closed up the nursery they had lovingly created in their home for an adopted baby—promised, but never delivered—David described grief that descended like a tsunami wave, slamming him to the bottom of the sea. He could not do much more than lie down and blankly watch through underwater eyes as his life-dream dissolved away. Our therapy sessions were full of tears. I could offer little advice as we cried together over the pain of dissolution. Was this therapy, I wondered? Would healing come of our time together? He paid me to be fully present with what I had learned about therapy over the past fifteen years of my career, but all I could do in the beginning was join him tearfully in the suffering of such an elemental loss.

I had resources from which to draw in Jungian analytic psychology, as well as in developmental and clinical psychology. I knew plenty of interventions to relieve David's pain and help him redirect his life. But something stopped me from intervening. What was it? Though I cared for David and wanted to help, I had a strong sense that if I were to do so I would actually prevent something essential from being born. Neither of us knew what that might be. We had to trust walking into unknown territory together, see what there was to see, and respond to what we found. At first this felt like standing in empty space with no compass, since we did not know what we were looking for. But we met each week, and eventually David found comfort in being with me in the therapy room itself. He could be just as he was: miserable.

In my office were shelves of objects that could be used to build and tell stories, much like children did when they played in a sandbox or on the beach. My sand tray, which was twenty-four inches by eighteen inches, was a place where worlds could be created in miniature. The perimeters of the tray provided a symbolic container for David during this time of dissolution, giving him a chance to explore what had been invisible, but was pressing from within. We looked at his dreams and watched the sand tray stories he made to represent his grief. What emerged from the worlds he created were scenes of stepping out from behind a glass case into the natural world, where music was bountiful. As he traced his fingers in the sand, David told me about his love of gardening, how he longed for the summer months when he had time to dig and turn the earth and do the planting that always brought a sense of peace, much like meditation. But here it was midwinter, gray, stark, and cold, with no possibility for gardening for a long time to come.

Several months into our work together, David brought in a small terrarium of tiny indoor plants to show me. He had planted them with tender care, arranging the tiny live world just as he had done in creating the symbolic sand tray worlds in my office. I could see a little bridge over pebbles, suggesting a trail through the woods, and bits of moss and bark to simulate the flora of this miniature forest in a bowl. Turning toward nature gave David the first bit of pleasure he had experienced since falling into his depression. Over the next few sessions he would tell me of the changes that were happening in the terrarium, and how the tending of it had become like a daily devotion. Eventually he had to transplant all of it into an old fish aquarium, not only because of prolific growth, but because he wanted to experiment with putting in a system for running water.

The little terrarium took on a life of its own, eventually requiring a fairly large space in David's house, but there was nowhere to put it except in the closed-up room of the old nursery, a place he avoided. After packing up and removing all the baby's toys and clothes, the crib, changing table, and dresser, David had locked the door. At first that felt right to him, but over time the closed door actually pulled him toward the room he no longer called a nursery. He did not call it anything. The room was simply empty and he had wanted it that way. But his avoidance had turned to its opposite, becoming instead a tangible force pulling him towards the room. Tentatively, he decided to step inside to see what happened.

He raged, down on his knees, furious at the immense, heart-felt effort over all the years, the persistent, unwavering pursuit of his dream, the forgiveness, and continuous trying, again and again, but all of it for naught. Why? What meaning could there possibly be in such failure? Why was it that others could have children with next to no effort at all and not even want them, when he and his partner were ready and willing, yet refused by the gods? He could not accept such a cruel fate. When his ranting turned to tears, he finally just lay down in the middle of the room, exhausted. Upon awakening, David knew that he would go into the room every day for at least an hour until he figured out what to do with it.

In the beginning, he brought only himself and a pad of paper and pen to catch whatever emerged in the silence. Then he moved in pillows to sit on; then he did not go in for awhile, but soon found that he missed the room. Being there satisfied some urge he did not even know he had. Eventually he moved the terrarium in for company, which by then had a moat of water around it. Plant life thrived, along with a plethora of snails. David found himself humming whenever he tended the miniature world of nature. He installed a water pump and made a little waterfall, adding fish to the moat; then he made the moat larger until he had created both a live underwater world and a live forest world to view at the same time.

We both recognized that the nursery was giving birth to something new in David. He repainted the room and moved in a rocking chair and table. He began to meditate, but did not stop humming. Sometimes the exhalations he made resonated with sadness, other times with joy, and still other times they were like a chant or a prayer. Sound-making became his healing. Like a musician practicing scales, David practiced breathing sounds at different pitches. He let music flow through his body as though he were an instrument of his own breath. This daily devotional not only helped to heal his broken heart, but it brought forth a gift to share with others.

One day, David spontaneously made songlike sounds while sitting with a friend who was terminally ill. The friend described David's voice as a link with the divine. It helped her feel a bridge of hope spanning the worlds between life and death. Others also began to recognize this emerging new gift in David and invited him to share his healing chants with people who were moving through all kinds of life passages, marriages, divorces, births, and deaths. He was discovering a true vocation beyond his career as a schoolteacher. He let it inspire and guide him into the next sanctuary of his own home, then into a world of healing sound as a sanctuary for others. David's genius was a continuously regenerating gift for self and other. With the help of nature, he had stepped into the vulnerable heart of healing, where he found a most surprising and unexpected resource to share with the world.

CHAPTER 13

Alchemy of the Present

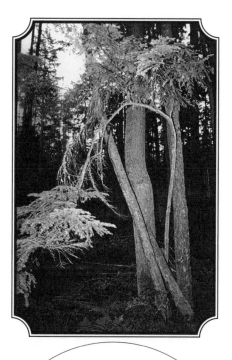

Responding to the Present
has found a unique solution
in the competition for sunlight amidst a cluster of trees
growing closely together.
Rather than growing upward, it arched
into available sunlight with its topmost branches lowest to the ground.
Langley, Washington.

Chapter 13

When my vision opens beyond its own preconceived patterns of reality, I am able to see and learn from the essence of what is before me. The word "essence" comes from the Latin *esse*, meaning "to be; that which makes something what it is." Trees, for example, reveal their life stories in the shapes they take. I can sense the essence of their lives by observing them as they are growing in the present, or I can see them according to their names, classifications, and history as a species. By opening our focal lenses to understand more than what fits into our patterns of thinking, we are more likely to perceive the essence of a moment or the convergence of moments. By tending to the verb of the matter before us, we can experience in an embodied way what is truly alive in each moment. Synchronicities and creativity thrive in such moments.

The word "matter," which we think of as the substance that things are made of, evolves from the Latin *mater* (mother). Its meaning is clearly related to the word "essence." Both are of the feminine, whereas *pater* (father) and its derivative word "pattern," meaning "form," are of the masculine. I view the space between the masculine and feminine, the pater and mater, as the place where creativity is sparked in the present. It is where something new can be born, or is alchemically produced through the pressure of opposites. I call this in-between space *liminal*, from the Latin *limen* (threshold), fitting into neither the masculine nor the feminine pattern, but encompassing all possibilities.

I consider the soft-eye focus that one must have in the practice of yoga to be an actual example of how to perceive, or be in a perceptual liminality, an in-between space. It consists of the polarities of stretching and releasing, bending forward and backwards, all the while breathing steadily and deeply. Though one's concentration and presence to the moment must be profound while moving through the postures and breathing, one cannot prefer one polarity over another. Rather, the practitioner of yoga must be able to experience fully the body's opposites while not identifying with them. One must stretch, make effort, while also relaxing and breathing. If one pole is preferred, there is no possibility of reaching liminal space, the threshold through which one might experience the divine. It is a rare phenomenon in time and space to be in a state of motion, but not to move toward or away from one pole or another, rather to be simply and completely present for a moment of life. Such thresholds are the spaces where synchronicities are more easily perceived, where creativity is more likely expressed.

Healing with nature has provided me with the opportunity to experience this liminal place between pattern and essence, and I consider it a sacred collaboration to share this threshold with others. It requires both doing and being as well as the soft-eye focus open for discovery. The interactive field between my clients and me is considered a *temenos* (safe place) for welcoming the soul to manifest itself in the world. In the true sense of the word "collaborate"—to work together—we create this *temenos* together. There are always two with authority in such a process. We both learn from and teach each other, no matter what developmental stage the client is in when therapy begins.

I believe that all healthy relationships involve a desire to learn and teach. This is true between teacher and student, client and therapist, spouses, colleagues, mentors, and between parent and child. In a generative parenting process the child must be able to teach the more powerful parent how to respond, and the parent must be willing to learn from and respect the vulnerable in order to become an effective parent. As the parent is responsive to the child, the child learns to be responsive to both self and other. By learning, the parent naturally teaches. This, too, I consider to be a most sacred collaboration.

During a visit with friends who were raising nine-month-old twins, I noticed their primary parenting style was in making their babies safe to discover on their own. They witnessed, responded, interacted, but they also left plenty of space for their children to learn what they could do and how they could be. With this freedom, they were more able to initiate confidently into the world. Depending on a child's stage of development, the parent would of course provide more or less guidance, but always the parent must be willing to learn from the child as well as teach him. There must be an attitude of discovery between the two distinct polarities of parent and child for creativity to come forth. In the creative process there is always a collaborative learning and teaching phenomenon going on within the artist. This could be called the will interacting with desire, or the ego with the self, or power with the vulnerable. There is a profoundly important relational experience going on within when the inner call demands a response: the desire to sing and the song, a need to move and the dance. A flow of energy needs to be moving between the poles.

A professional dancer who was a client of mine asked me to work with her in the studio as she prepared to choreograph much of what she had learned in the previous three years of our work together in the office. She was most concerned about finding the right relationship to her art, her family, clients, and to herself during our psychotherapy work. The dance she was in the process of creating had to do with her emerging vision of art as life, not separate from life. She included her children in a portion of the piece expressing cycles of birth, life, productivity, old age, and death. My role as therapist in the studio with her had to do with witnessing, seeing with fresh eyes, acknowledging the flow between her ego and self, the two poles that provided the liminal space for her creative process.

It was important for my eyes to see her in this process as part of integrating what she had learned through our creative collaboration in the office, as well as to witness her much later in the public performance of her dance. Ordinarily, I did not attend my clients' public performances or shows, unless doing so would have a particular and positive contribution to the therapeutic relationship. Part of the reason for this had to do with time constraints. I also wanted to make certain that the therapy was not confused by a duality of roles. This meant always clarifying that even out of the office, we were not in a social relationship or one that benefited the therapist or client outside the business contract of therapy. Whether in the studio, office, walking in nature, or meeting clients in their homes, the purpose of the encounter was on behalf of the client and creating a safe space, a *temenos*, in which healing could occur.

Another dancer, a thirty-year-old man, asked me to witness the performance of a dance he had choreographed about dying, grief, and rebirth. Since much of our work in the office had to do with his learning to survive, then finding another way to be in the world after his father died, it was essential for him to experience completion of this healing process through the manifestation of dance. My presence was an integral part of the articulation of his newly integrated being, something he could not have translated in dialogue sitting across from me. I learned more about him by watching him in artistic motion than I could have in a year of dialogue within the office.

In another scenario, I had discovered the necessity of scheduling a session in the home of a client whose brother had died recently. I did so because opening the urn which contained his brother's ashes was not something he could have done in the office, yet he very definitely could benefit from therapeutic support. After we shared the hour together in his home, I understood what a blessing it was to witness my clients in their own territory, away from the office. I could experience them in their power as well as their vulnerability, thus encouraging the flow between the two polarities within therapy. So often clients and therapists focused primarily on the wounds in therapy and did not have a chance to witness also the strengths.

This was certainly true for the client who had adopted a one-year-old child from China and wanted to celebrate the manifestation of her lifelong dream. But to continue her sessions with me she would have had to leave her son with a babysitter, something that would have not been therapeutic for either of them at that time. She had been taught that the bonding between adoptive parent and child, particularly as a single parent, could not be interrupted during the first several months. Also to be considered was the need to establish a safe, consistent, and familiar environment without introducing the child to too much that was culturally foreign. On behalf of what was beneficial to my client's continued therapy, we agreed to meeting in her home. Though the hour progressed quite differently than usual, my witnessing her interaction with her baby at home helped solidify her new identity as a parent.

Another client, with whom I had worked for many years, wanted to change the form of our therapy so she could move from problem-solving to a more liminal place of discovery. During our eight years of therapy together, she had come to terms with having been sexually molested as a preadolescent girl. She had also finished college, found a job that suited her, dealt with an elderly parent's illness, and bought a house. She successfully ended her therapy feeling confidence in herself and the life she had created. A year later, she returned and asked me if we could do another *kind* of therapy. She did not feel a need to focus on problem-solving anymore. She wanted to explore her own creativity but did not know how to begin. Honoring the alchemy of the present, which nature's language had taught me so well, I responded to her call.

She wanted to move out of the "problem-solving chair" but was not sure that was possible. Together, we decided to experiment by rearranging the chairs in my office. Many things happened through this joint collaboration besides creative inspiration. We pulled my chair across the room so it was beside the toy shelf, and we moved her chair into the center of the room so she could gaze either out the window or at the toys. This gave her practice in the soft-eye gaze, not concentrating on problems to fix. She discovered a more spontaneous self-expression when not studying my face and my reactions to what she said. I realized she would benefit by the kind of witnessing I gave my client the dancer, but this time the witnessing needed to go on in the office, not the studio. Our work together during the previous year of honoring the call and response provided a prototype for what needed to happen within herself now. She wanted to practice in front of me, to be witnessed in her newly emerging process in a predictably safe *temenos*, one she had helped create and had learned to trust.

Since my own healing with nature had created new vision in me, I could now see that finding new life in the office was also happening, that it was not just about walking with clients, nor was it just about learning from nature together—rather, it was about seeing, combining, embracing all differently. Therapy was for me a sacred collaboration, a true and inviolable working together. As I let myself discover what was before me like I had with the trees, and be *response-able* to what I perceived, I felt fully present to what was called for in the moment. Though therapy was often called the "talking cure," talking was not always what was needed. An energy flow must be alive between therapist and client for something to happen, whether or not words were being exchanged. I had learned there would be a profound relational experience going on within, if there was also one occurring between client and therapist.

My desire to help, understand, and articulate could sometimes stop the flow of understanding between my clients and me, when what was called for had to do with not words, but energy. Noticing how the energy moved and stopped within our therapy had provided one of the best barometers for how effective therapy was at any moment in time. This was when something was happening, coming alive in the space between us. Practicing *notitia*, as I did with the trees, simply noticing what was occurring before me and within, required full presence to the exact moment I was in with another person. *The alchemy of the present.*

When one of my clients, Matthew, would begin to sag and go limp, almost curl forward in his chair during some point in our dialogue, I would respond with empathy, which always surprised him and brought him back into the present with me. Such sagging proved to be a familiar state in his life, a fading away from the present moment, a giving up on himself. When we were able to trace back from those sagging moments in the office, we discovered that he was responding to an internal voice, an advice giver, one who spoke to him as *you*, directing and planning or discouraging him. He rarely had an opportunity to simply enjoy the state of being with his desire. No wonder he would sag forward, feeling always driven beyond himself. By experimenting together we also learned that it did not help to *answer* back to the internal voice, because he would usually lose the argument. Instead, he tried going to the soft-eye focus that one must have to enter the liminal state. By doing this he learned through the images that came to him what his true desires were, before the intervening voice could talk him out of them, redirect, or refuse to hear him. The pictures were more powerful than his words, though they often presented images of his vulnerability. They were a more accurate expression of his feelings than his words had yet been able to translate. When we both paid attention to the images he created, his energy would come surging back into his body.

With him I felt like a scout on the trail, traversing an inner landscape rather than the actual outdoors. The internal journey presented an equal amount of wilderness to explore side by side as the walking therapy had done with other clients. I was able to use much of what I had learned in both places. He helped remind me how vital it was to be in a joint discovery process together, to not acknowledge what wanted to be noticed before he could discover it himself. Like a scout, I was more experienced in exploring the inner wilderness, but I needed to know where he wanted to go. I could walk metaphorically beside him, experiencing my authority while inducting him into his own.

I also learned, by staying tuned to energy flow in the interactive field, that some dreams needed not to be interpreted, or understood or related to in any other way than to be present with the dream's experience. I learned this the hard way with a client who had looked forward all week long to sharing her dream with me about flying into a most unusual and unknown territory. As I began discussing the possibilities, looking at the elements of the dream, the dynamics, the storyline, the mystery being revealed, I noticed her increasing agitation. It seemed so incongruent to the dream, which I felt had a very positive message for her. As she squirmed in her chair, I found myself trying even harder to translate for her. The dream seemed to be a gift of joy to a client whose primary difficulty at that time was an overly stressful life with no room for play or rest. Her dream stepped in and gave her a lift.

I could not understand her resistance to my interpretations, until finally she became quite angry with me and said all she wanted to do was share the experience. It had been such a thrill in the middle of the night, but she had been alone then. Now, she wanted me to enjoy the dream with her. That's all. Simple. I had missed the point of the dream by not being responsive to its message in the moment: to authentically share the experience of joy. When we acknowledged that her anger at not spending time with me that way was probably how she felt much of the time within herself, we could move into the next truth about to emerge. Responding to her anger provided a model for her internally developing interactional field, so essential to the healing and the creative process. She needed to develop a speaker and a listener within, not a lecturer who overrides the audience with a speech. And I needed to remember again to be present without preconception.

Treating the healing process as if the unconscious always needs to be made conscious, or something broken needs fixing, or a problem needs solving, did not ring true in the practice of therapy as a sacred collaboration, as an alchemy of the present moment. This process was more aligned with the creative process than with the medical model of therapy. Using nature as a guideline, when a branch stretched itself across a boulder to grow laterally rather than straight upward, it did not mean it was in need of anything other than making use of all the resources it could find for furthering life.

CHAPTER 14

Healing with Trees in the City

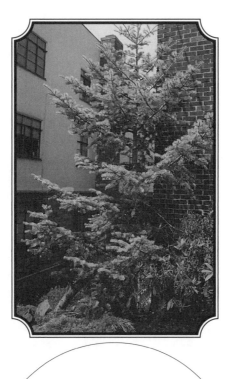

Facing the Wall

started out life growing at a sixty-degree angle that only
righted itself within twelve inches of hitting the wall of an apartment
building in the Eastlake neighborhood of
Seattle, Washington.
It turned to grow alongside the wall until it could surpass the roof.

Chapter 14

Walking down the sidewalk toward my office building, Lana was always relieved to see the large cedar tree that marked the path leading up to the front door. She often touched the reddish-brown trunk when she turned onto the path, finding that her body began to relax no matter what the stresses of the day had been. After a hectic week, followed by a near-meltdown in rush-hour traffic, Lana once told me she felt like she had stepped into an oasis as soon as she passed under the cedar boughs. The green of the front lawn, completely encircled by hedges tall enough to give a sense of privacy and sanctuary, also offered the sensation of time slowing down for her to finally reflect and hopefully heal from cyclical depressions. Nature always welcomed her.

We had been doing walking therapy sessions for several years. She preferred walking to sitting in the office, and we both looked forward to checking on the familiar living touchstones that grew along our forty-five minute walking route. Lana sometimes noticed a spontaneous reflection of her own process in the trees, but on occasion I asked directly what pattern of growth she perceived in a particular tree we had been watching over time. One of her favorites was a blue spruce that had been growing along the outer wall of a two-story apartment complex. Finally, the top twigs of the tree had reached the roofline that overhung, blocking any further upward growth of the tree. We were both curious to see how the tree would negotiate this obstacle in its path. Lana thought it would bend and find a way around.

I thought it might do that too, but another possibility was for the tree to send its life force into the lower branches to become fuller and more lush than tall.

Noticing its early growth a year before, Lana and I had stood in front of this blue spruce tree, marveling at the creativity that followed what could have meant disaster at the start of its life. The base of its trunk leaned at a forty-degree angle for the first six feet, heading straight for the apartment building. When it reached within twelve inches, it must have sensed the immovable object in its path, and turned radically at a ninety-degree angle to proceed growing straight upward for the rest of its life. We guessed that it had been growing for about twenty-five to thirty years altogether, keeping a perfect distance of twelve inches from the wall. Now, it had reached the ceiling and was a beautiful tree, all branches thick with healthy blue needles.

Both Lana and I had recognized the parallels of this tree's life to Lana's early life, and the radical turn she had to make for survival. Her childhood had been marked by profound boundary violations within her family to which she been unable to stand up. Avoidance was her best defense, but left her too isolated for thriving. When her parents divorced, destabilizing the whole family even further, she turned toward the consistency and structure of her parochial school as an alternate family. The school and the relationships she developed with other caring adults served her well, just as the strong wall of the apartment complex had served the turning tree. Now here we were, years later, watching the tree's life in the present as it reached the ceiling, about to outgrow the wall altogether. I wondered what Lana might imagine was similar between her and the tree now. I could not help noticing that our walking therapy had become focused almost entirely on her current issues; no longer was much attention given to her past. I asked her directly what she was thinking about as we stood in front of the blue spruce.

She laughed and said, "This sounds like a Rorschach test!"

Though I do not use this kind of diagnostic test in my work with clients, Lana, as a well-educated psychotherapist herself, knew it was a psychological test for assessing projections. In other words, what a patient imagined in an unidentifiable image, or inkblot, would be indicative of the patient's mental state. It is a way of turning outside what is going on inside, with the hopes of understanding what is driving a person's behavior or thought process.

I could not help laughing with Lana about looking at our blue spruce as a Rorschach.

"Actually, I'm interested in more than your projections," I answered, as we continued our walk along the route we had walked so many times before.

"I know. Let me think about it for a minute."

We walked in silence for a few blocks, both of us letting the rhythm of our bodies guide the rhythm of our thought process. In the quiet, I found myself counting a walking mantra that matched my steps, left-right, left-right, like this: Na-ture, Rhy-thm, Stor-y, Soul-pause. Though I did not consider it a song, exactly, the rhythm felt naturally soothing and inspiring. Creative ideas often flowed more freely within the syncopation of these words and my footfall. Walking beside Lana, I found myself thinking of how our reading the signs of the natural world along our city walking route felt more aligned with the Aborigines' song lines, than the Rorschach test's projective images.

The Aborigines made songs of all they observed along their walkabouts, describing lizards and clumps of plant life, hillsides and animal tracks, changes in soil, mud puddles, stones holding precious water. The words to their songs became musical maps of a territory that had no trails or maps to follow. Whenever they met another walker, they would each sing the songs of where they had been, translating the upcoming territory for one another, the rhythm of their songs reflecting each person's walking rhythm. When I had asked Lana to tell me what she was thinking as we stood in front of the blue spruce, I wanted to know what she actually recognized or discovered in the tree's pattern, and what she recognized in herself. Though our relationship to nature could offer a reflective mirror, a generously neutral place for projections to be made and more clearly understood, I felt it offered a vastly more complex set of gifts than this. Being in and with the natural world allowed what I called *entrainment* to a more healing rhythm than the machinations of the city.

The literal meaning of the word "entrain" is to become like a train, to share the track. It is most often used with musicians, particularly with drummers who are jamming together and discover a common beat or a rhythm that carries them all along. Babies held close when they are upset can calm themselves by entraining to their mother's slower, steadier heartbeats, and women who spend much time together often unconsciously synchronize their menstrual periods. Patients who are placed side by side in preparation for surgery have been found to share a natural entrainment with one another's heartbeats, revealed by similar electrocardiographs. For people to harmonize with their environments is a natural tendency. Walking in the natural world within the city helped us entrain to a very different rhythm from the hustle-bustle of downtown traffic's frenetic pace, allowing our bodies to find our right music as we walked and talked side by side, as Lana and I were doing.

Lana had been having her creative thoughts in the silence too, and I was eager to hear what she had been pondering.

"Back there with the blue spruce, I realized that I don't always see myself as flawed anymore." She smiled, "Not that I'm flaw-free, just that it's not the first thing I think of."

"You're not feeling so depressed these days, are you?"

"Well, it's summer, and that always helps to have the sun, you know. I think I'm in pretty good balance with the meds, and I've been walking everyday, watching my diet. It all counts. But the main thing is I'm thinking differently about things, not so critically first off."

I too had noticed these changes taking place in Lana over the last year or so.

"Remember how I told you I didn't want to do cognitive

therapy because it had never worked before in my other therapy?"

I nodded.

"When we look at the trees, I cannot think in the same old patterns. My mind doesn't go along the old repetitive pathways of my brain. I have to think differently. So perhaps we've been doing some form of cognitive therapy all along."

I said, "You're probably right. Our eyes are intimately connected to our brains. The way we see makes a huge difference in how we think. Maybe we've been doing a form of *EMDR* without even knowing it."

EMDR is a psychotherapeutic intervention akin to hypnosis. The eyes must follow a pattern of movement without moving the head while thinking of a traumatic event that continued to be fresh and hurtful in our memories. The hope was to reprogram the brain to respond differently to the previous harm, so we could move ahead without endlessly repeating the thought that causes reinjury in the replaying of it. Learning to use our eyes differently not only changed our perspective, but also the patterns in our brains. When our eyes are filled with the natural world, it is hard to keep repeating internal negativity either subliminally or consciously. Lana said she could not help but notice something more positive in herself than flaws when she stood in front of the blue spruce, watching its valiant effort to reach as high as it possibly could in spite of what had happened to it earlier in life.

Though Lana and I had been walking the same neighborhood route for a long time, it was only recently that we noticed the powerful life force of a maple tree lifting up the sidewalk around it. Was this because it had so recently happened or because our eyes opened to it when we were ready to see how it paralleled a struggle Lana was having in her life? Perhaps it did not matter. We were simply able to find meaning and inspiration in the continuously evolving touchstones in nature as we did our walking therapy together. Sometimes she noticed a change and sometimes I did. This kind of *notitia* felt to be a form of play, another welcome healing force in Lana's therapy, and a sign of her continuing movement toward health. By "play" I did not mean lighthearted or not serious; rather, I meant natural and spontaneous, with humor.

Contemplating the maple tree with Lana one day, I remembered being surprised that we could be laughing about what we had before cautiously and carefully identified as an annihilating, critical inner voice that had kept her imprisoned away from life. We had worked with this voice from a variety of different perspectives, including antidepressants, until I finally said in exasperation, "Just don't go there anymore. It's not telling the truth about you!" But it was not until she noticed what the maple tree

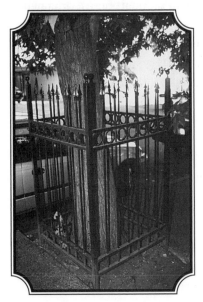

was doing with its life force that she took it to heart and was able to at least confront her inner imprisoning voice when it tried to deflate her. She had to see a living image in order to substitute for what her imagination repeated time and again. She needed something more tangible for this change to matter.

Encircling the maple was a three-foot-high wrought-iron fence around its base, which was originally meant as a protection to a young tree in the city. Now that it was at least forty-five years old and had a sturdy trunk of at least sixteen inches in diameter, this tree no longer needed a wrought-iron

149

Beyond Protection, *growing within the wrought iron fence of a Seattle city resident, and having many of its upper branches cut to make way for telephone wires, this tree's roots have made more room for itself by buckling the cement of the surrounding sidewalks.*

protector. The tree had become so powerful over the years that its roots lifted up the sidewalk around the edges of the fence, buckling the cement four inches off the ground. Because it grew under the telephone wires, the tree's upper branches were routinely trimmed, forcing the growth to go down lower on its trunk and into the roots. Peeking out through the bars of the encircling fence, a new sprout of growth was growing close to the base of the tree. It was seeking sunlight from under the sheltering umbrella of the main trunk.

It was clear to us both that the wrought-iron fence was now a jailer of this powerful tree, sprouting new life above and below and lifting up the city sidewalks to make more room for itself. In comparison to the life force of the tree, the fence lost its power as anything more than an inconvenient, unattractive ornament, irrelevant and cumbersome at best. Lana liked seeing her own imprisoning fence in a similar light, laughing for the first time at its stiff, rigid repetitions.

Chapter 15

Synchronicities: The Art of Nature

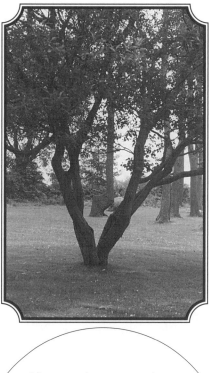

Nature as Art *creates a picture*
of beauty
with the frame of its branches (in foreground) at Chetzemokah Park
in Pt. Townsend, Washington.

In the background is a tree that was likely covered
early in its life and had to find another place to grow from.

Thus the crook at base.

Chapter 15

*S*ometimes I go about in pity for myself, and all the while a great wind is bearing me across the sky. This Ojibwa saying marked a real turning point for me. During the first few years of struggling to heal and make meaning of it all, I oftentimes found myself absorbed in lamenting my fate, not celebrating the great wind that might be carrying me exactly where I needed to go. Little by little, I began to accept the possibility that my back injury had cracked me open to another way of being in the world. All my relationships and perceptions were affected by my changing vision of life, death, and regeneration. I thought about my friends, family, colleagues, even my writing and photography in relation to these cycles of life in nature. No longer able to see with my old eyes, a surprising synchronistic event occurred to affirm this fact.

I received a roll of film back from the developer completely double-exposed, with babies floating across each frame into the sky. My partner and I had just spent the weekend at a bed-and-breakfast and had not seen any children at all. We wondered how our film could have been processed with someone else's. It did not make sense at all. In the very last frame, a close-up of the child's face was superimposed exactly over mine so that my eyes were looking out through hers. In the background, floating in the sky, was my stepson's smiling face gazing into the baby's. We deduced that he had loaded our already-exposed film into his camera before racing off to take photos of his infant niece's christening.

We had a composite of our different experiences framed within one photograph. Two worlds at once, a synchronicity. The word "synchronous" breaks down to mean "occurring with time": *syn* (with) and *chronous* (time). I knew there was no causal connection between the photograph of myself with eyes of a baby and the changing perceptions that were clearly occurring in my life and my work. But there was without a doubt a link that could not be explained. I called this a "pearl of coincidence," and enlarged, framed, then hung the photo over my writing desk. Healing with nature had cracked me open to seeing with new eyes, like a child who learns from all of life. From that moment forth, I began to celebrate the *great wind that was bearing me across the sky.*

My whole life was affected by this changing vision. While I had been tracking the transformations in my work with clients, I had not noticed how completely the rest of my life had been transforming. With the youngest of five children finally off to college, my partner and I had shed city life and moved to a more rural part of the Olympic Peninsula. We found a house overlooking Discovery Bay with an expansive view of the snow-capped Olympic Mountains in the distance and Protection Island, a bird refuge, in the near view. Many evenings at sunset, we sat on the porch to watch deer grazing in our front lawn, eagles soaring over-head, or raccoons emerging

153

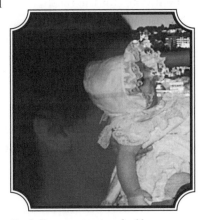

Fresh Perspective *is a double exposure of me with a child's face superimposed over mine. My eyes are looking through hers, symbolically seeing life from a new perspective.*

from the storm culvert under our driveway to make a fast break for the cedar grove behind our house. In springtime we watched as the wobbling backside of a baby raccoon tried to catch up with its parents, who had already disappeared into the trees. Then another one wobbled past. And another one still. A family of five altogether. We were delighted to be on their map and we fully supported the neighborhood covenants which protected freedom to roam for all wildlife.

We had landed in a nature-lover's paradise. Even the commute to Seattle, which reminded us each week of the huge price we had to pay for paradise, was worth what we came home to every single time. No matter how weary I was at the end of a week's worth of work crammed into three intense days, I always felt thankful to step out of the car and look up at our celestial treasure of sky uninterrupted by city lights. The stars shone like scattered jewels on black velvet. We always bypassed our house for the beach, no matter how late we returned home at night. Soft sounds of water rolling beach rocks along the shore, with wind rustling through Madrona trees on the bluff, became essential antidotes for the harsh, constant, grinding buzz of city life.

The natural world continued to offer its inspiration beyond the healing of my body and beyond the emerging new vision of my work, and I continued to write of the synchronicities. Gradually, I realized there was more to this story than discovering new vision in psychology. Something more mysterious and compelling drew me to look beyond the journey of a wounded healer. It was certainly true that in healing myself I had learned what would be helpful to others, and that my work as a psychotherapist was greatly enhanced. But the story that was unfolding did not end there. I kept listening and looking for the clues and signs of life around me. Living close to the elements in Pt. Townsend made such openings all the more nourishing and bountiful.

One evening, as I lounged on the deck overlooking Discovery Bay, I was surprised to see a lone dog sitting in the open lot across the street, completely still. Unusual for a dog to be loose like that in this neighborhood because a strictly honored leash law protected wildlife. Also unusual for a dog to sit frozen like a sculpture staring up at me. I just looked back, fascinated. Behind her, the sun was just beginning to descend over the mountains, casting a gold shimmer over the water. With no warning, not even a twitch of an ear, she leaped up and pounced deep into the high grass. Only the long, fluffy plume of her tail could be seen waving in triumph.

Flushed with the thrill of this rare moment, I slipped away to find my camera. Never before in my life had I seen a fox in the wild. Here she was, hunting right in front of me. Thrilled, I felt my body tingle. She must have watched me long enough to ascertain that I was no threat to her or her feast. Even before I slipped quietly back onto the porch, though, I knew she would be gone. Survival depended on it. As long as I was a known factor, on my porch, far enough away, and not moving toward or away, all was well. My mistake was leaving the moment to capture it with my camera. Though disappointed not to have more time with her, I considered my lesson. Stay present, see what I see. Be changed by the offerings.

The fox reminded me of the opportunity I had been given to feast with my eyes and my heart in this new home of ours. No matter where I looked, I recognized a real story in the natural world as fascinating to me as any fictional account of the extra-ordinary. This viewpoint filtered into my creative writing, revealing another way my vision had changed in healing with nature. All it took now was being in the present moment and opening my eyes. The stories flowed forth, like this one I wrote about the neighbor who had lived and died in the house across from ours:

My neighbor's windows looked to have tears leaking from their edges last night as the sun set over the bay, gold spilling across the water. Fred died in March. It was the middle of June, and I could not forget this man I had not even met. The dark windows in his house stared like empty eye sockets, haunting me.

From my deck across the street I tried not to look back, but in the spring I watched his rhododendrons, daffodils, and tulips stretch to the sun. They bloomed without him. I was grieving a man I did not know, a man who lived alone, had no family, kept to himself, and died of a massive heart attack while on holiday. Another neighbor told me this two weeks after he died, or I might never have known. Since moving to the neighborhood last fall I had only seen Fred twice before and from a distance. He wore a plaid shirt under bib-overalls while pruning his apple trees. Before he left for his holiday I saw him again, dressed the same. He was leaning on his rake, laughing and talking with a neighbor. This is all I knew of Fred.

But in knowing this, I imagined odd conversations with him, saying things like, *What a surprise to die when you're in the midst of things, when life continues as if you'll return. Your dark green house that needs a new roof, your apple trees, and all the blossoms in your yard; your stunning view of the bay, your red and white pickup truck waiting in the driveway; the neatly stacked woodpile at the side of your house; your satellite dish busy collecting information; and those lonely windows. Oh, and there's the woman who drives a car with California license plates. She has come to mow your lawn again. She tends your yard as if she likes what you've left for her. Soon other cars from different states park in your driveway. People carry things out to their cars. Eventually pieces of your life drift away with them, easily, like petals in the spring breeze. The woman continues to tend your yard. I think she's living in your house now. Painters come and move your old pickup from the driveway to the roadside. They change the face of your house from dark green to gray, but the windows still look sad.*

I only thought about Fred when I looked at his house from mine, and always with a deep lament. That is, until the day I walked on the beach in front of our houses and almost stumbled across a dying seal. At first I thought it was just another log washed to shore, but when I smelled the stench of decay and noticed the flies swarming on its blood-caked, patchy skin, grief surged up and stopped me cold and shivering. But the seal snuffled, and I could see mucous running from its nose and mouth. He was breathing ever so slightly. My god, he was still alive! Maybe I could do something. I turned and ran home as fast as I could, panting into the telephone receiver when the sheriff's department answered. I had found a dying seal on the beach at Discovery Bay and please come quickly. Maybe we could save his life.

They put me in touch with the Marine Center and I described what I had seen, trying to calm down. The specialist asked me too many questions I could not answer. What shape was its head; how long were the fins; how much fur on its body, or was it smooth-skinned; were its fingernails at the tip or midpoint of its fins; did I see its teeth? After all those questions, I felt I had not seen the seal at all. I was perturbed by the delay. Why was the marine specialist obsessed with these details? Why not just rush down with a veterinarian and see for herself? Do something to help the sick seal! Patiently, she explained to me that this was the season for elephant seals to molt their skins. Since Discovery Bay was so peaceful, they often chose that beach to go through their week-long transformation.

I wondered if my presence had disturbed the seal, who already had enough to do as it was. But the specialist asked me to return to the beach and check on all the details she had asked about, and call back to let her know if indeed it was an elephant seal. I returned with my camera.

The beached seal, whose colors blended with the gray and black of wet beach rocks, the soft tan of driftwood, was actually hard to find again. Having run for help so quickly, I had not made note of his location. He was no longer there. He had turned himself all the way around and was snuffling painfully across the rocks and barnacles toward the water. Miraculous, I thought, relaxing now that I understood this process to be a molting, not a dying one.

As the tide came in he heaved and struggled inch by

excruciating inch towards the water on his little fins, resting every few feet. When he finally reached the water's edge he rolled in, letting the waves wash him off. Then he turned and labored ever so slowly back across the rocks, up to his molting place. Drying in the sun, scraping along over the rocks and sand, rolling in the ice-cold waters—all contributed to his essential change of skin. A metamorphosis before my eyes. I was reminded of how painful change is, no matter how essential it may be for survival.

Honoring his privacy, I turned and headed home just as three fawns walked across my path. I watched them tiptoe along the rocks to the bay, then wade in the water up to their knees. Two of them very carefully backed out while the other squatted and peed in the water. I laughed and they all turned to look at me, huge ears tuned like radar. I photographed them, too. Through the lens I could see a splash of scarlet on the hillside above the fawns. The red rhododendrons in front of Fred's house waved, making me look again at his house with the empty windows. But I felt joy, not sadness, as I experienced the gestalt of that exact moment with the fawns standing before me, the seal molting behind me, the flowers blooming on the hillside above. I honored the rhythm of life with its mysterious, continuous cycles of celebration and grief. Transformation was in the air all around me. And within.

In the past I had relied mostly on psychology and art as my touchstones, my guides through difficult passages. My career as psychotherapist and writer depended on them. Yet over the last few years of my healing journey, nature had become the altar to which, like a spiritual devotee, I returned again and again. My eyes had changed. I saw through nature's lenses a way to travel beyond the familiar myth of the wounded healer. Through myth and story it seemed that psychology could recycle and reframe, but could not reveal a new pathway. I had previously relied on the generativity of art to balance the limitations I found in psychology. But I was beginning to understand that the natural world offered more than a balanced perspective. It had become so compelling and insistent in my life that all I could do was turn toward the force that pulled me completely into the present. See what there was to see, and *let the great wind bear me across the skies.*

CHAPTER 16
Poetry of Walking

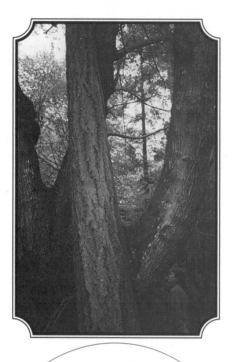

Helpmates,

a pine and a maple,

provide each other with extra stability by leaning into one another

as they grow on a steep hill

in South Whidbey State Park, Washington.

Chapter 16

My friend and colleague Francis incorporated walking into his schedule so that it would be easy for us to get together and do walking consultations. He and his wife Kyla lived in Poulsbo, about an hour and a half from Seattle via ferryboat. We would arrange to meet for consultation at the ferry dock in downtown Seattle, then walk along the waterfront to Myrtle Edward Park and back. Our first hour would be spent talking of professional issues, but within our second hour, walking back to the ferry dock, we often covered our personal lives too. Francis had been trained to diagnose pathology and prescribe treatment for his clients, though he had questioned that pattern of thought for many years. He had decided to further his training in Jungian analytic practice as I, too, had done, hoping to expand into a more holistic way of perceiving the healing process.

We shared the idea that people had an innate drive toward health, and that psychotherapy did best when it helped clients find a connection to this instinct within themselves. I told Francis about seeing this as the same force that made it possible for trees to create radical turns in their lives to reach more light. He agreed, and said this often meant giving our clients space to find that light, rather than crowding them with too much treatment. He was concerned about the particularly vulnerable clients who came to him already feeling identified with being ill and disabled because of previous treatments that had so labeled and treated them. Francis felt that certain kinds of therapies invalidated the spark of life that needed safe space and a little fanning to ignite for the client to make real change. He tried, as I did, to stay away from diagnostic terms and judgments that might limit our clients. We both felt discouraged by our profession's lack of creativity in conforming too rigidly to preconceived notions about pathology and treatment.

As we strolled along the shoreline of the park I recited my walking mantra: Na-ture, Rhy-thm, Stor-y, Soul.

He laughed and said, "Ah. The poetry of walking. Soul-walking."

I smiled and repeated his diagnosis of what I had been doing in my own healing process, then sharing with my clients by way of walking therapy: The poetry of walking; soul-walking.

I told him about my trip to England and what I had discovered on the Wayfarer's walk through the Cotswolds: that what I had been writing of the pilgrimage into nature was about more than my own and my clients' stories of healing. My wayfaring companions from all parts of the world had awakened me to the obvious: that nature's gifts were available to everyone who was open to them. I pointed out to Francis how we were doing our consultations afoot. Soul-tending our clients and ourselves. Creative sparks were flying everywhere.

I said, "I've decided to take note of what happens between people and nature, not just about the psychotherapy process."

"You're going to write about your friends, aren't you?" he asked with a smile.

"Of course. Families too. Colleagues. Whoever wants to be included."

"I don't mind," he said, humming my mantra, Na-ture, Rhy-thm, Sto-ry, Soul.

We could hear the water slapping up against the rocks along the waterfront, seagulls calling nearby. The sounds lulled us into a peaceful reverie as we both felt the conversation shift into our personal check-in time. We asked one another about our families. I told Francis how much living in Pt. Townsend reminded me of where I had grown up in Tucson, Arizona, with its wide open spaces and surrounding mountains. Though vegetation and climate were radically different between the northwest and southwest, I found a similarity, a sense of being at home, whenever I was close to Puget Sound, with the Olympic Mountain Range on one side and the Cascade Mountains on the other.

Francis told me how much he and Kyla enjoyed living in Poulsbo, a ferryboat ride away from Seattle, directly west. They had a view of the water that reminded them of home in Hawaii even though the northwest climate was as different from the tropics as it could possibly be. We wondered if our senses of *being at home* with our lives might have more to do with feeling happy at midlife than being on the water. Francis laughed and wanted to share an epiphany he had recently had about his twenty-year marriage to Kyla. All the while he had been circumnavigating the globe, gaining ever more training and education, looking for spiritual mentoring and magic, as well as the right livelihood, the most significant and essential teacher he had was actually living at home with him. Francis, still amazed by this discovery, went on to say how grateful he was they had managed to weather all storms together and still be on the same ship, happier than they had ever been in their lives, both individually and as a couple.

"Wow! What's the magic key that opens that door?" I said.

Very humbly, he said, "We are truly lucky."

"For sure." I was well aware of the extraordinary challenges they had faced together, including the unfathomable pain of losing a child. Many couples cannot weather such a loss.

"We both feel like the other one was there in support and love like no one else in the world could have been. At the exact right moments of making or breaking it in life. Early on, I helped shore up Kyla's foundation. We got together twenty years ago, just after her divorce, when she was trying to work and take care of a two-year-old. I had my career already launched and was wanting a family. When I had to make a radical change in my career a few years ago, she was there 100 percent, even when all was at risk. I needed that kind of support more than I ever imagined. I had to learn to surrender. Kyla showed me how to do that and keep my self-esteem. Best spiritual lesson I've ever learned."

He went on to tell me about Kyla's new career as a life coach, and how proud he was of her stepping out into the world with such confidence after raising a family. In some ways they were changing the dance of their marriage. He now enjoyed being able to relax more at home, while she was thrilled about developing her career, interacting with colleagues, and being more fully engaged in the world of work.

As Francis described how his life was now flourishing beyond all expectations, I knew the exact trees I would photograph and send to them as celebration of their twenty-year marriage. A Douglas fir and maple, about forty to fifty years old, grew within each other's arms along a path called the Hobbit Trail in South Whidbey State Park. They actually looked like they were dancing together. Fate had placed them right next to one another, in just such a way that when the maple looked as though it might fall downhill, one of its lower branches merged into the trunk of the Douglas fir and was able to find enough ballast to continue its upward growth. Years later, they came together again. This time the trunk of the now-sturdy maple offered strength and support for the long, lean fir tree to lean into it, thus providing security against the ferocious winds that had ripped off the tops of many surrounding trees.

There were spaces in their togetherness, as Kahlil Gibran describes in speaking about marriage in his book *The Prophet*. In psychological terms they were an individuating couple, standing in their own uniqueness, learning to accept and love their differences, talents and limitations included. They merged at essential times in their lives, but they had not created a fused or codependent relationship. Both were flourishing and able to live fully into their own truths while also creating a beautiful dance of love.

Coming together, coming apart. Ebb and flow. All natural rhythms of life. Just thinking of life as a dance of rhythms, like my dream had suggested several years previously, had been one of the most helpful puzzle pieces to understand. It helped me not stay attached to my judgments about relationships staying together or coming apart. Often, space was essential for thriving, especially within relationships that might already be too merged. I told Francis how I was trying to use this mode of thinking to accept and reconcile my sadness over the coming apart of the relationship between my sister and brother. Though both lived within miles of each other and also my parents, they no longer spoke to one another. They had split apart into a silent standoff that was upsetting to the whole family, particularly my elderly parents. Everyone was still in shock, not clear about what to do.

A serious argument and mutual misunderstanding caused them both to strike out in outrage, leaving them both feeling rejected and profoundly hurt by the other. Neither was willing to be in the same room with the other yet, much less speak by phone. Both wrote letters and both complained vehemently to everyone else in the family. But an angry silence persisted between them. After hearing the story from each and every family member, fortunately or not, I understood how the story told about the crisis, though different for each, was the certain truth for each teller.

Until recently they had been completely involved in each other's lives, with spouses and children providing an active extended family. Both couples were present and had helped with the births of their children, sharing childcare when needed, and all the family holidays with my parents. Since I lived in Seattle and was busy with my five stepchildren, I was only able to share in these gatherings every few years. Still, all members of my family considered us to be a close-knit clan. Though my elderly parents at first hoped I might be able to help mediate with my skills as a therapist, I recognized early on that I could not do therapy with my own family, though I tried at first. Finally,

I recommended they each see a professional counselor either separately or together, if they could.

They both did this separately, but sadly it did not lead to reunion. While reciting this story to Francis, I thought about the essence of sharing. Though the telling may not change anything in fact, having our stories heard and received sympathetically makes all the difference. This is what I offered each family member, no matter how many times each of us might need to lament our fates. And Francis offered this to me, listening without comment or judgment, while I turned the crisis over and over again, always looking to see if there might be something else I could do to help, besides pray. Then he asked very quietly, almost shyly, what kind of similar situation might I imagine in nature. Touched that he wanted to use my own medicine on me, I mentally thumbed through my file of tree photographs, but could not imagine an existing situation that reflected wisdom for my family.

"If you could let go of this crisis being only tragedy, I wonder what else might be there," he said, inviting me into doing what is called *active imagination* in Jungian psychology.

I imagined a cedar grove with five main trunks, all strong and thriving, as each of my siblings, my parents, and I were doing in our own lives. From a distance all trees together sculpt the shape of one large cedar tree, a family. If we were to step into the grove of my imagination we would see interconnecting roots, sprouts wanting to branch into the light, but the sheltering trunks do not have enough room between them. They are too close. A cataclysm occurs, possibly an earthquake, creating an opening in the grove. Eventually, a stream flows through the crack in the earth, light streams in. Creative new life forms around each of the five main trunks, extending the grove across broader territory.

Without judging it, just looking at the results of my brother and sister's refusal to be with or talk to one another, there was in fact space, more clearly separate territory between families within the larger grove. Was this a plus or a minus? It was not what any of us wished to happen, nor did it reflect the family values we had learned to live by. We as a family were in unknown territory. Time would have to show us all what might come into the open space. None of us could know beforehand. The only choice seemed to be in how to look at and live with what was not going to change anytime soon, if ever. I recognized that we could no longer enjoy having the whole extended family together, but must visit each nuclear family separately. Beyond the obvious heartache of this, it seemed to be defining and differentiating the individual groups that made up the family, much the way I imagined would happen within the cedar grove when the cataclysm opened more space for the light to filter in.

I glanced at Francis. "For now that's the best I can do with my imagination."

He gently assured me that he felt certain there was just such a story incubating right now, somewhere. And when I came across it, perhaps it would help to bring my family for a visit.

Amazingly, Francis's blessing came true in its own unique and surprising way years later. The creative sprouts I had anticipated growing more fully into the metaphoric space I had imagined with the cedar grove after its cataclysm actually happened by way of the grandchildren.

As my brother's and sister's children grew up, they knit together with their love, vitality, and sense of humor an interlinking network of roots and branches that now sustains the whole family. I have six nieces and nephews who have matured into very distinct, wonderful people who have figured out how to love unconditionally each other and all of us *old folks* in the midst of an ancient family cataclysm. They live in present-time, so the split for them is simply past tense. They insist on new territory, and we are lucky they care enough to show us all how to step into it.

CHAPTER 17
Breaking Open to God

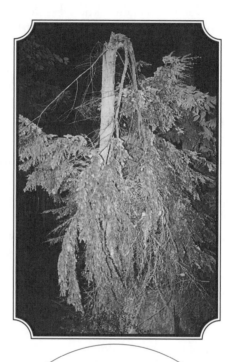

Breaking Open

had the top of its trunk broken

so it dangles from what looks to be dead bark, but it continues

to thrive both above and below the break.

It has lush foliage shaped more like a bush than a tree now.

Langley, Washington.

Chapter 17

My friend Angie was diagnosed with breast cancer at age thirty-three. She had been married fourteen years at the time of diagnosis, was the mother of a five-year-old daughter, had completed her MBA in finance, and had worked several years previously in the university comptroller's office. She told me that the moment she heard she had cancer had been a paralyzing shock, but by the time she reached home, she knew for certain that all significant aspects of her life would be radically changed forevermore. She just did not yet understand how. Seventeen years after that diagnosis and all that followed in the years of remissions and recurrences, Angie was able to tell me how her life and every relationship had been altered, like lightning shattering the top of a tree. From knowing herself as a steady, certain, stable person, Angie's encounters with ten bouts of cancer and its treatment had turned her into a woman whose common denominator with life had become constant change.

One of the most poignant responses she remembered hearing after her first diagnosis was her mother saying, "This can't be happening to you. You are our rock."

This was how Angie had always seen herself as well. Her role in the family had been to bring the equilibrium back to center point, providing a sense of balance within the whole family. Even after she was married and had started her own family, Angie continued to play this role in life, not knowing any other possibility until cancer cracked her open to the continuous changes required of her. In reflection, seventeen years later, she considered the date of her first diagnosis to be the beginning date of the person she had become. Who was this person?

Angie told me that she had turned toward the call of spirituality. Jesus Christ became the primary guide for her life. This developing relationship evolved over time through extraordinary health difficulties and the heartache of facing the continuous losses in her life. Within the past four of the last seventeen years, this relationship has led Angie to knowing and being her fullest self. She told me that almost every waking moment had become lush and abundant with a complete presence for life and whatever happened in it. Like the tree whose broken top prevented it from growing any taller, Angie's life had become profuse with a most powerful and generous life force in all the branches below the break. Angie was a woman who lived fully with cancer, and her life inspired others to embrace their sense of God as fully in whatever ways they might be called to do. This was not proselytizing, but living simply and opening to each and every moment, of turning toward life rather than away from it, whenever the choice was presented.

Such choices were presented to Angie each time her cancer recurred. The shape of her life could be seen in her responses to those choices, as difficult and painful as every single recurrence had been for her, her family, and her friends, beginning with the very first. Not atypically, Angie's first doctor considered family history, statistics, trends, and treatments protocols, rather than the actual person trembling before him, desperately worried that the lump she had felt in her left breast might be cancer. He unfortunately tried to laugh off her worries, saying that because of her age and lack of family history, she could not possibly have breast cancer, that it was more likely a cyst. He suggested she return for a follow-up check in six months. Tragically, he said the same thing six months later. But when a friend of Angie's died of breast cancer, she went to see another doctor and asked for a biopsy. No one was prepared for the biopsy to come back positive—least of all Angie, who had hoped to rule out cancer. She had wanted to alleviate the concern that her body could not let her forget.

The first major turn toward life Angie made in that moment was to begin trusting her own body over other people's opinions or theories. This turn saved her life several times over. In the whole journey of cancer treatments, Angie was the only one to have detected any of the recurrences, the first being three and a half years later in her lymph nodes. Her close connection to her body had allowed her to detect even the slightest changes and be able to read whether the alterations were benign or not. When red streaking showed up on her breast, she insisted on a biopsy in that location, though the doctors said there was no indication of a recurrence there. The day after the biopsy the streaking mysteriously disappeared, and the biopsy revealed a malignant mass. There was no medical explanation for this, but Angie had come to understand that her body communicated in whatever ways it could. Now she immediately responded, sometimes awakening in the middle of the night with a clarity of vision that always proved to be true. Such responses made up the new shape of Angie, a woman who no longer served as a rock for others, but as a thriving, continuously changing inspiration for how to live more closely aligned to our own lives and our own bodies.

Her expectation of doctors and the medical system had been transformed over the years, from believing that they could save her from the devastation of the disease to recognizing that the system and people in it were both brilliant and limited like all humans are. By finally being able to look toward God for the only *saving* possible, she was able to find forgiveness for all human errors and shortsightedness along the way, both in herself and in others.

The way she put this to me was, "I have found unbelievable peace and acceptance of the circumstances through Him, not

Him through the agony of the circumstances, but a work in progress."

Angie also told me that as her spiritual connection intensified, so did her sensitivity increase to the beauty and wonder of nature, whether it was in the way light slanted across mountains, the phenomenal Arizona sunsets, or hiking down the Grand Canyon. She perceived all of nature as a demonstration of God's creativity and healing power.

We were in high school when I first met Angie. Her best friend and mine were sisters, so we saw quite a lot of one another on family vacations and in school. During a recent Christmas we all happened to be in Tucson together and we planned a reunion luncheon. Amidst laughter and tears, we shared a diversity of life experiences, discovering that each of us had turned toward some form of spiritual practice, something none of us had expected to do when imagining our futures in high school. Though our lives had been very different from one another's, no matter what the obstacles, each of us tended to turn toward the light, each of us in our own particular ways. But Angie's spiritual life had accelerated the most of any of ours to the point of becoming her full-time vocation, not only in all she did, but within her leadership role at church as well. She had always been active and productive, raising her daughter to become a successful adult in her own right, owning her own franchise business, being fully active in community, church, schools, and nonprofit organizations. But cancer had made her realize that her energy and attention would be minimized by the demands and side effects of treatments, bringing about the conscious decision to eliminate activities and responsibilities that did not involve serving God in some significant way.

Over the past seventeen years Angie has survived and thrived beyond the first biopsy, followed by a lumpectomy, radiation, chemo; a bilateral mastectomy and reconstruction several years later, more chemo and radiation; then a bone marrow harvest, hysterectomy, more chemo; bone and liver lesions, radiation, and still more chemotherapy. I asked her to describe to me the significant turns she had been inspired to make in her life as a result of these recurrences and their excruciating, almost annihilating treatments. The most difficult by far, she told me, was learning to let go of the people she loved and allow them to live their own journeys through life. Since her vision had been cracked open so completely, she understood how little time there was to waste in not being present. She recognized that most people did not share this perspective because they had not had to face so directly the possibility of a shortened life. Honoring everyone's unique sense of urgency and even their oblivion to life and God was her biggest challenge. She said she only became fairly successful at this over the past four years, when she made a full-time commitment to her spiritual calling.

Coinciding with this commitment, Angie had discovered in her body the presence of bone and liver lesions. Though her immune system had been able to heal some of those lesions with the support of chemotherapy, new ones continued to appear. Each member of Angie's family faced these devastating facts in very different ways. Angie finally had to come to terms with the fact that her family was more oriented to making external adjustments in response to cancer, whereas she had been devoted to making internal adjustments, of becoming more of who she was meant to be. Finally accepting these disparate perspectives had helped her make the most significant turn to date: to live and let live. To truly let each person become whomever she or he was meant to be, just as Angie now recognized herself to have become her full self by living through the challenge of death again and again, only to find a closer relationship to God and life at every turn. She told me that this relationship had blessed and brought more to her life than she could have achieved on her own.

She offered this quote by A. W. Tozer: "God rescues us by breaking us, by shattering our strength and wiping out our resistance."

In return, I sent Angie a poem I had written in honor of her brushes with death that had so clearly brought her fully into life. The title of this poem, "Relampago," means "lightning" in Spanish. Another Spanish term is in the poem: *duende*, meaning brush with death. The surrealist poets of Latin America believe that brushes with death, the *duende*, are a gift to one's creativity because it breaks down the barriers that keep us from seeing the beauty of the divine.

"Relampago"
When lightning ignites your life, shattering all beloved
structures that held you so well, securities and comforts
now smoldering to ash, do not wail, do not curse the gods
for such an unexpected fate. Remember the Duende.
Remember how Spanish poets fall to their knees praying
for a brush with death, for relampago to burn away veils,
so they might, for only one brief breath, inhale God.

When lightning's jagged edges rip through your life,
Leap like Lorca, from your split and shattered tree. Break,
finally, from any confines of your imagination like Athena
from the skull of Zeus. Sail into each wild storm, quaking,
but always toward the duende. There, you'll find gold
on the legs of a honey bee, lacy wings sturdy enough
for flying to where tears, only of gladness, dwell.

The *duende* can also be experienced through letting old ways of being in oneself and in the world die away. Gary, an artist friend of mine, did this by choice at the height of his art career in New York City. When he realized that he was living a false life by exploring only the dark side of things through art, he knew he had to let it all go. Gary knew something central was missing from his life, but he did not know what that might be, only that he could not continue along the path he was walking. By his own will he broke the top off his career by destroying all of his art, closing his studio, and ending that chapter of his life. Then he cut himself loose from all securities and comforts and every familiar structure in his life, no longer working, no longer eating, no longer in an intimate relationship, no longer in his home. He wandered and was silent and celibate, like a monk on a fast. He soon discovered that he must find God or die. This search became the central principle around which any life he was to live from that point forward must be constellated. It was the only life he wanted, yet he had no idea what it would look like or how he might find it. He simply decided to do nothing until he was moved by some sense of God from within. Trusting that he would be shown, guided, or inspired by the life force in some way, Gary decided to wait until such connection was made to proceed in any direction with his life.

Many of Gary's friends, and certainly his family, worried that he might be having a nervous breakdown, or in psychiatric term perhaps a psychotic break. What others thought at that time in his life, though, did not matter to Gary, who was a strong, healthy, intelligent, and artistically talented twenty-eight-year-old man, who wanted passionately to live his most authentic life. He knew no other way to change tracks from what had felt like a false life to a genuine one than to let go of what he had created completely and irrevocably, to really let his old self die away, and pray for the real self to manifest in its own truest form. His only certainty was that God had to be central to his life. Over the next ten years Gary wandered without creating any art and without working for money. Like a mendicant, he accepted the kindness, generosity, and shelter from others, always giving something back of his own innate generosity.

Inadvertently, but instinctually, he practiced what Lewis Hyde wrote about in his book *The Gift*. Hyde defined the gift economy as being natural to native peoples living close to the land and depending on a barter system, a sharing of resources. Keeping gifts circulating was primary to such a system. Gary relied on this economy, even though he was a modern man living in a high-tech city. He was a survivor, learning how to live differently as he walked through unknown territory, developing skills he had never imagined possible. Naturally endowed as an artist, he could use his hands and his mind to figure out how to fix, create, rebuild just about anything that was needed in the homes of the people who offered him shelter. Rather than seeing him as a burden, people experienced Gary as a welcome addition in their homes. Most of life for Gary had become focused on being and trusting that God would be revealed in all situations and circumstances. As he developed a strong and certain primary relationship to God, it became clear that another call awaited him beyond existing close to the margin in New York City.

In 1988 he moved west to Whidbey Island and became associated with a spiritual community, Chinook Learning Center. Gary's talents were warmly received immediately by the

people he met, especially a woman who worked there, Alexis. She was both educator and song master, her voice beloved by all who heard her sing. A creative artist in her own right, Alexis had also dedicated her gifts to furthering spirituality rather than commerce. She had completed her master's in Spirituality and Culture and was facilitating workshops and groups as part of her work with Chinook Learning Center. Gary and Alexis became close just as her life took an unexpected, cataclysmic turn that surprised the whole community. Alexis's husband of twelve years suddenly left Alexis to marry one of her friends. This turn came with no warning, no process, no time to do careful transplanting of their relationship.

The shock and trauma quite literally blew the top off Alexis's life as she had known it, sinking her into despair. Gary stood by as her friend while she knit her life back together, slowly but certainly, over time. He was not afraid of the depths of darkness and death that traumatic losses could bring up for a person whose life as she knew it was suddenly shattered. He had already walked that path himself and had not only survived, but thrived. He held the faith that she would also thrive. His belief inspired

Alexis to eventually find her own new life force within and begin to blossom again. After a few years their friendship evolved into a more passionate love, and they decided to make a life together. They had found a natural and easy rhythm of being with one another, even as different as their backgrounds were. They began to create together.

With Gary's building skills, Alexis was not only able to maintain her house, but together they could fulfill the dream of creating a retreat center within their home. Gary began painting and making sculptures again and was delighted to discover that his images were more joyful, inspiring, and playful than they had been in his NYC phase. With Alexis's support he found a way to bring his art into the world of healing and spirituality rather than the competitive world of commerce. Gary continued to practice one of the first things he had learned after destroying his art years before: that anything given with love circulated and became generative. Gary's art would soon be found in many people's homes, but not one painting or sculpture was ever sold. He offered his art as gift, hoping that it inspired others to feel closer to their own authenticity and sense of God.

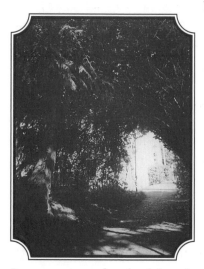

Passageway *is an arboreal arch formed by the creative collaboration of a quince bush and cedar tree growing over a sidewalk in the Eastlake neighborhood of Seattle, Washington.*

Eventually Gary and Alexis married, bringing together a large gathering of friends to celebrate their intimate commitment, as well as their devotion to doing spiritual work as a couple. Together they facilitated ongoing dream groups and spiritual practice with music and art, inviting participants into their home and onto their land so they might experience a closer connection with the natural world as part of their spiritual devotion. Their coming together had proven to be as generative as the forest that surrounded their home. They sheltered and inspired whomever came into their lives, reminding me of an arbor formed by a quince tree and a cedar. Though both had to break open at a certain point in their lives to find one another, their branches had eventually intertwined to form an arbor passageway. A blessing for all pilgrims passing through.

Wounded Healers Collaborate

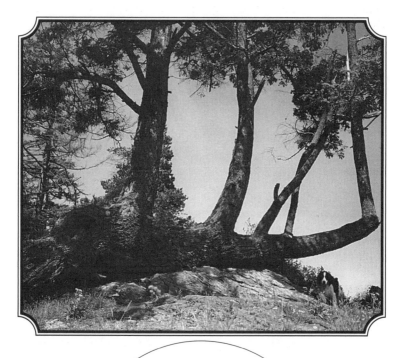

Community *grows along the ground*
near Orcas Island, Washington.
Ferocious winds likely blew this healthy tree to the ground,
but it thrived by becoming ballast to the five branches that transformed
into trunks.

Chapter 18

Many of my colleagues considered themselves wounded
healers, as I had also done, and created life work in their healing
process. But Annie, a yoga teacher, never intended to make a
living from the practice that had saved her from living a life of
chronic pain. As a young woman she intended to be first a
professional athlete, then a social worker. She had the perfect
body type, size, and musculature to make her dream of becoming
a star gymnast very real at age fourteen. But a serious injury
changed the course of her life. Annie had been performing on
the parallel bars, her specialty, when she found herself very
suddenly on the floor, flat on her back, unable to breathe and
unable to move. She thought the fall had knocked the breath
out of her so completely that her lungs had collapsed. Stunned
and paralyzed, movement was not possible. Breathing was
paramount. It was not until she had been x-rayed at the hospital
hours later that the doctors finally diagnosed three broken
vertebrae in her thoracic spine, which had made breathing near
impossible. She was very grateful the damaged vertebrae had not
been in the cervical or lumbar spine, which controlled
movement of arms and legs. But the pain was so severe and the
panic over not breathing so all-consuming that Annie knew she
was in a fight for her life.

Though surgery was considered to alleviate Annie's pain, the
doctors could not guarantee that it would make any difference.

Forty years ago, prognosis for successful back surgery was never certain. It often brought about further disability because the back muscles, so essential for supporting the vertebrae while they healed, would be severed during surgery, thus causing two injuries to heal. Annie and her family decided against it, but nothing else she tried gave her any relief from what was fast becoming chronic pain. Rather than focusing on her dreams of soaring as a young woman, Annie was absorbed in how to get through her days without being too debilitated or distracted by unrelenting physical suffering. By the time she was ready to graduate from college, Annie could no longer tolerate such a life of pain.

One morning she awoke with a very clear thought. Unless she could recognize a sign that very day that there was another way to live, she would end her life. Proceeding through her day in a fog of despair, Annie walked into a bookstore to return some of her textbooks and discovered her sign from the gods. The only title she saw in the entire store that day was: *Yoga for Bad Backs*. She bought the book and read about how she might find both pain relief and a spiritual practice to help her create a new life. Immediately, she contacted a yoga master to work with and experienced enough natural attunement with the practice to take a significant turn in her life. Finally pain-free, Annie began working full-time as a social worker, fulfilling one of the career dreams she had had before her back was broken. Continuing to study at the Integral Yoga Center in New York with Swami Satchidananda, she soon discovered that what she had at first thought was a supportive spiritual practice became central to her life. By then married and with a child, Annie became a yoga teacher herself.

Three years later, she was diagnosed with an ovarian cyst that was suspected to be cancer. Again Annie was inspired to learn another way of healing. Though her doctor insisted on surgery, Annie had developed a certain level of confidence in her capacity to heal naturally. She wanted to try as many health alternatives as she could in the hopes of curing it herself. She fasted and drank powerful herbal teas, used clay packs, meditation, hands-on healing, and kinesiology, and within a month the cyst had disappeared. This second miracle of healing inspired Annie to study alternative healing methods at UCLA experimental college, where she learned about polarity balancing, metaphysics, hands-on healing, and the gifts and visions of psychic practice. Annie only knew that she was hungry to learn as much as she could about the natural forces of healing in both the physical and emotional realms.

When she and her husband divorced after twelve years of marriage, Annie drew on all the self-healing skills she had learned to create another channel for her life force, as she had done twice previously. Because she was a single parent, Annie's income from teaching yoga had to be supplemented, so she began to take on students who wanted to learn about psychic and hands-on healing. She became known and well-respected as both yoga teacher and healer on Whidbey Island, Washington. Annie inspired me to try yoga again, something I had avoided doing because of my back injury. I had reinjured my back several times by doing forward bends incorrectly, so I was very cautious about any kind of exercise that might distress my lower spine. But when she told me about having healed her own back injury through yoga, I decided to give it a try.

After class I described how I had been healing from my back injury by walking in nature, learning to see my healing process in a way that was inspired by the generative force of the trees.

"Oh," she said, "Maybe you'd like to see my meditation tree, then."

We walked to the hill behind her yoga studio, where she showed me a large tree that was lying fully on the ground from the base all the way to the top of its trunk. It looked as though it had been growing like this for a long time. We deduced that it had fallen many years previously. What would have been branches on the tree had become separate tree trunks in their own right, tall and abundant, flourishing with life overhead. It seemed perfectly natural for the main trunk to be horizontal on the ground to provide stability and nourishment for those branches to transform into trunks. It had found a way to create several lives in one, just as Annie had done after her life-changing fall.

Annie said, "Coming to this tree for my morning meditations is one of the things that helped keep me going after my divorce. I prayed that I would find the creativity to make another life for my son and myself. And we did it," she said proudly. "Now that he's grown up and living his own life, here I am back at the drawing board, ready to create still another one for myself."

I said, "Well, here we both are, two healers collaborating on the twists and turns of fate, trying to understand the meaning of it all. I find this midlife time such an interesting period because we've lived long enough to have created and recreated our lives several times by now. "

Annie said, "Besides, swapping our stories is fun. Reminds me we're not in this alone."

We were easily and naturally cross-pollinating our healing talents as wounded healers, while nature helped us make the bridge.

Several other friends and colleagues whose careers were shaped by the wounded healers' journey also shared their rich resources for healing self and other. Sylvia, trained in naturopathy, had healed from her asthma through the natural remedies of plants, instead of relying solely on Western medicine's steroids and inhalers. She made herbal and homeopathic remedies for herself, patients, family, and friends, always with her eyes and hands attuned to what was growing seasonally in the natural world.

I remembered walking around Green Lake in Seattle with Sylvia and another therapist friend, Marty, who was apprenticing with a Chinese herbalist in the hopes of healing a chronic skin condition. As we walked and talked, Sylvia's attention would tend toward the ground foliage, whereas mine was more focused on the shapes of the trees. Marty walked between us with descriptions of the Chinese Qi-jong energy work she was learning. At one point, Marty laughed at Sylvia and me when she noticed that our body types and our perspectives seemed to match where our attention to the natural world and healing was directed. Sylvia, at five feet, four inches tall, was closer to the ground, whereas I seemed more aligned with the tallness of the trees, at five feet, eleven inches tall. My eyes looked upward to see the stories that inspired my thinking about healing, while Sylvia tended to what was on the ground. She noticed the different species and what they offered homeopathically.

As we shared our stories, cross-pollinating our different fields, I wondered what happened when wounded healers healed.

Sylvia answered, "Well, I sculpt with clay."

Marty said, "I dance."

I wrote poetry. It seemed that we as healers continued to follow life's generative urge wherever it was needed, whether into healing, creating new philosophies, or making art.

My friend Bill, who was a psychosynthesis psychologist, wrote poetry and created conscious, sustainable community in his retirement. His call to become a wounded healer had come in early childhood, when an accident cost him the use of his right hand. He was only a year and a half old when his hand was caught and mangled by a baker's mixing machine, causing him to lose three of his fingers. For most of his life, he experienced either no sensation in his right hand or random pain. He became an expert in working with biofeedback, a systematic way of retraining the brain to relax when under stress or pain, so as not to cause the body more pain. After a successful career in psychology, Bill was able to retire by the age of sixty-two and focus with his wife on building a new community with several other families who wanted to live in close connection to the natural world.

Wounded Healers Collaborate

Bill and his wife Mary bought land together in Colorado and collaborated in creating an intentional community that would be supportive and nurturing through their retirement years. His career as wounded healer had naturally evolved into being a creator of new worlds. This turn coincided with a major surgery he opted for in which his right hand was reconstructed over a long period of time. Though his childhood injury had been one of the events that had set the course of his life as a wounded healer, the surgery and his retirement marked how he had come full circle. The surgery involved a series of steps which culminated in grafting his right hand onto his own side for six weeks while the tissue and nerves grew into his hand, giving him the physical sensations he had been missing since his childhood injury. More essentially, the surgery finally alleviated the random pain. This made it possible for him to use both hands in all the building and woodworking that he was now devoted to doing as community-collaborator in his later years.

I, too, felt the call to collaborate within community after my healing was complete. My back injury had finally healed after close to five years of tending it, listening and learning from it, changing the way I lived on its behalf. I walked daily, but was also able to kayak and do yoga, ski and backpack, activities I thought I

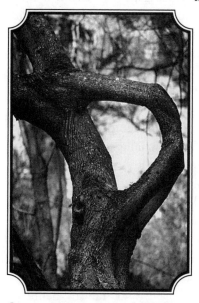

Connection *grows in South Whidbey State Park. What remained of a broken branch found an ingenious solution to high winds by circling back to the main trunk to make an enduring connection.*

would never be able to do again. As a wounded healer who had finally felt healed enough, I had a passionate urge to create within community, so I applied for admission to an evolving community of learners and teachers who practiced Jungian analysis. I was delighted to discover that my work with nature's healing process was warmly received by my colleagues. Jung himself had compared *individuation* to the growth process of a tree—after all. I felt great kinship with this new fellowship of colleagues.

Our evolving community was dedicated to making room for the creative contributions of each of the seven candidates who were preparing for the practice of Jungian analysis. For the next four years we worked on integrating and articulating what we learned from the rich resources of seminars with analysts from within our community, and with visiting faculty from all over the world. We participated in colloquiums to discuss our work with clients, the books we were reading, ideas related to *Jung's Collected Works*, and the practice of Jungian analysis.

We studied a variety of other clinical modalities of psychotherapy as well, though most candidates were already well-grounded from many previous years of education and clinical practice. We met regularly with mentoring analysts who, like artists of the soul, supported and challenged each one of us to find our true voices and articulate truth as clearly as possible, both in writing and in verbal discussions. Supervision of our work with clients and personal analysis was at the heart of this community of healers. I had found my true professional kinship group. When it came time to make a formal presentation of our creative contributions, I gathered all my tree photographs, selected twelve with the clearest messages of healing and regeneration, enlarged them to poster size, and framed them. My presentation involved inviting my mentors and colleagues to wander through this gallery of tree photographs so they might have their own first impressions before I described the stories and how they intertwined with the human transformational process.

The title I chose, *Nature's Alchemy*, fit with what I wanted to translate of what Jung had written on ancient alchemy and the process of the human quest for wholeness.

Jung had compared individuation to alchemy in that persons who embarked on this journey had a similar metamorphosis to go through, stage by arduous stage, from lead to gold, or from being unconscious to becoming more aware of how one interacts within one's self and within the world. Nature's transformational process revealed a live, present-day form of this philosophy of alchemy. I believed nature's offering would add something valuable to the concepts of alchemy, thus expanding the philosophy from chemical metallurgy into the animate world of life.

187

One of the best examples of this living alchemy could be seen in the life of a tree I had come across walking around Green Lake in Seattle. Its main trunk had a hole in its center. One of the branches above this hole, in response to what may have been perceived as a mortal wound, reversed itself to drop straight downward as a root and grow parallel with the main trunk. This branch actually transformed its cellular structure, as in alchemy, rooted into the ground, then changed again, this time to trunk cells, so it could

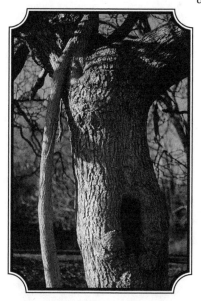

Crutch Tree *suffered a blow to its main trunk that has left a gaping hole. A higher-growing branch transformed into a root and dropped parallel to the main trunk until rooted in the earth. Then it transformed again to become an alternate trunk. Greenlake Trail, Seattle, Washington.*

provide an alternate trunk for the tree when the original trunk would die. In my opinion, this kind of alchemical transformation was as miraculous as metals changing from lead to gold. By studying present life through the transformations of trees, I thought we would not have to rely solely on ancient texts, past history, or psychology to find wisdom about individuation and the mystery of the life force.

CHAPTER 19
Life, Death, and Regeneration in Community

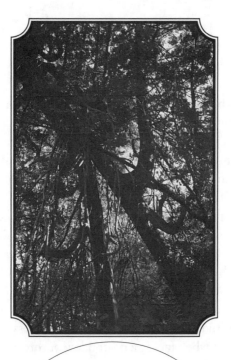

Split Tree *was pulled asunder*

by a mudslide on the trails above Golden Gardens

in Seattle, Washington,

leaving a ten-foot walkway between each side of the tree.

Yet it continued to live, changing branches into trunks

so that it was balanced against

the downward lean.

Chapter 19

Designed to be an evolving community guided by, and responsive to, each individual's quest for wholeness, the group of Jungian analysts I had joined with warmly received what I had brought to share from my discoveries in nature. They challenged me to go ever deeper into the source, which my mentors called "psyche" and I called the "life force." Alchemists, devoted to the long, very difficult process of turning lead into gold, named their work *opus contra naturam*, meaning "a master work against nature." Alchemical texts suggested that without intervention of the alchemist to help nature along, transformations would not occur. In contrast, I believed that the parallel process of *becoming gold* in human terms was a valiant struggle *within* our natures, not against it. In studying the transformational process of trees, I had discovered that when facing a death blow or threat to their lives, it was within their natures to transform cellular structure in ways that were similar to alchemy. This happened in nature without the assistance of arborist, alchemist, or therapist, because it was a survival instinct to further life. Inanimate metals being transformed in an alchemical process do not have such an innate drive.

As we challenged and supported one another's ideas and grew together as a community, a mysterious alchemical process was beginning to happen within our group of colleagues. A series of autoimmune disorders struck the women, like a blight in the forest. All of us were devastated by the unexpected onslaught of illness, especially when one of our analysts, a fifty-year-old woman who had previously been vital and very active, was suddenly diagnosed with amyloidosis, a fatal blood disease. She was given less than two years to live but died within the year. Another analyst in her late fifties, also healthy and strong, was diagnosed soon after with scleroderma, a slowly debilitating, eventually fatal illness that causes hardening and scarring of the skin both internally and externally. One of my colleagues had to leave analytic training for treatment of breast cancer; another had fibromyalgia, an exhausting and painful inflammation of nerve fibers in the muscles; and still another colleague came down with sjorn-gren syndrome, an incurable rheumatoid condition. Frighteningly, my own body had begun to give me warning signs that I was in danger of becoming sick if I did not make some major change in my life.

191

Friends and colleagues in other therapy communities also reported a high incidence of autoimmune disorders: a well-respected middle-aged analyst, having been recently diagnosed with Lou Gehrig's disease, was almost completely debilitated, and expected to die soon; a young woman candidate died of breast cancer; another from colon cancer; an analyst from a heart attack. Were these traumatic illnesses among women analysts and candidates disproportionate with the population at large? No one was keeping statistics, but stories passed between friends, and I became afraid. But of what?

Suddenly, being a female psychotherapist seemed dangerous to one's health. Why? Or, was it simply living to midlife in a highly polluted world that was life-threatening to us all? Were men becoming ill too? In our community it was the women, five of them. What could I do besides ask these questions and grieve the losses? What was really wrong, not just symbolically or metaphorically, but really and truly seriously wrong, that so many healthy people were becoming profoundly ill quickly? Were we the canaries in the mine? If so, where was the poison seeping in?

What was the poison? Could it be stopped or changed? How? Were healers becoming sick from sitting for long hours, working with other's shadow material and spending too many resources and years of training to do this? Were we all just working too hard? Were things so bad that this kind of work was called for? Where were the answers?

I prayed. *Please show me the way to understand what I could offer in behalf of the life force.* Please help me see clearly. I did not know what to do, so I went to the trees. I spent a lot of time reflecting in sadness about the disease processes that had so suddenly struck in the Jungian Analytic Community. I grieved the losses that preceded and followed. When our program had begun four years before, there had been an enthusiastic fourteen analysts and seven candidates. Now there were five very tired analysts and two candidates left. Our beloved community was coming apart. With my own divided family, I had to imagine a story in nature to help me reconcile my grief, but with the wrenching split within our community, I knew the exact tree I wanted to visit.

From a distance, this tree in Golden Gardens Park looked like the entrance to an A-frame cabin. It grew along a bluff overlooking Puget Sound and had been split by a mudslide or earthquake years before. The earth had shifted at least ten feet, the distance between each side of the split trunk. Standing in the midst of this split, I felt like I was inside the heart of a tree. Its grain was exquisite even after so many years of exposure to the elements. I could not imagine how it could have survived the trauma of being rent in half from its roots to twenty feet up its trunk. But it had not only survived; the cedar had transformed into far more life than its genetic destiny had been programmed. Beyond the split it grew at a sixty-degree angle for another thirty to forty feet, from which all of its branches had looped around in resistance to gravity and become a series of seven trunks. Each of these trunks, growing side by side for the length of the angled trunk, had together formed the perfect shape of a whole cedar tree. What a persevering passion for life this tree had. Certainly it had something to say to all of us who wanted to survive and thrive beyond the tragedy of our splitting community.

Whatever was happening within our group had been cataclysmic, very much like what had happened to this tree. Though all of us tried to assess what had caused the damage, causal factors would be impossible to determine. Trying to assess them might even bring about more harm. What difference would it make to the story of the split cedar, for example, whether it had been split suddenly by earthquake or mudslide, or had happened slowly over time with the cliff side eroding downhill? It was still split and still thriving in a completely unexpected way. Better to spend time noticing what was actually so and what followed, than to try and fix blame. Most apparent after noticing that the trunk stood asunder was that seven branches were able to turn and transform themselves into individual trunks. Each one of those seven trunks worked in communion with one another to create the shape of a whole cedar tree. A massive one at that, providing far more life to the forest than if they had remained branches of one main trunk. The creative process had a mysterious way of working things out. But it certainly was not how any of us imagined our lives would turn when we all converged together to create a community four years before. Seven wounded healers were still creating and collaborating, whether or not we formally graduated or were proceeding with our lives and work in whole new ways. Each of us was becoming a strong, generative, and unique contributor of life. Who was to say that splits are always tragedies? The cedar at Golden Gardens was courageous enough to let its most vulnerable heart show and still carry on with the devotion of furthering its life force.

I visited a retreat center in Crestone, Colorado, to rest and walk, meditate, and be with the natural world as fully as I could be, listening and looking for clues to follow into the truth of my next step in life. Driving through the gate, I noticed in my peripheral vision a cluster of gnarled and beautiful old cottonwood trees. But it was several days before I walked the hundred or so yards across the field to really have a good look. The trees had drawn me because of their close proximity to one another at their foundation, and the great flourishing expanse at the top. Was it actually one tree with a double trunk or two trees with a merged base? I enjoyed this walk under a very blue southwestern sky, with a wide-open view stretching for miles across the plains and the mountains rising up behind me.

When I reached the deeply grooved trunks of the cottonwoods, what amazed me the most was not their trunks, but a strong circling arm of a branch about ten feet above my head. This branch literally made several right angle turns at precise points to encircle the other trunk, which looked as though part of its trunk had been diseased or injured. Part of it was dead and would have fallen away had the branch not encircled it. That was impossible, I thought, walking around both trunks to make sure I was not just imagining such a possibility. The branch was alive and thriving, as were both trunks, and yes, the branch had embraced the other trunk almost full circle, not just with one turn, but several over time.

I wondered what had inspired such a relationship. They were definitely separate trees whose foundations had merged early on. Both had risen into their own separate glories, leaning slightly away from one another. They might have split apart without the embracing branch. This was the first time in all the years of observing nature's stories that I felt I was witnessing something akin to a moral choice. Though I usually tried not to anthropomorphize my beloved trees, I could not avoid doing so with these. Why else would the branch have encircled the other, had it not been to offer assistance? The branch could have made any number of other twists and turns to find light. I could see no apparent reason to have grown the way it had, except out of altruism. It did not want to lose its friend, kin, or mate. I could not know what the relationship was between these trees—only that they were in communion. I also did not know the depth of

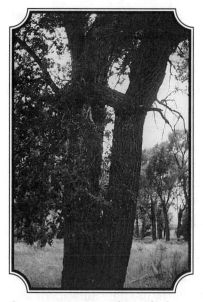

Communion *is a tree that evolved into two trunks, or two trees merged at base. The miracle is what happens higher up, after one tree started to die. A branch on the other tree circled around to hold it in place, until it created an alternate trunk from one of its branches.*

the lessons these trees exemplified for me, but I knew their message had to do with love. I knew I would accept their teachings wholeheartedly.

When I described these trees to a friend, he asked if I had heard about the set of twins who had been placed in separate incubators for the first week of their lives. One was not expected to live, but a hospital nurse fought to have both twins put in the same incubator. When they were finally placed together, the healthy twin threw her arm around her weaker sister in what looked like an endearing embrace. The weaker baby's heart rate stabilized and her temperature rose to normal. Our arms around one another, particularly when in our most vulnerable states, is a natural impulse of the life force. Good things tend to follow. Sometimes, even miraculous things.

Duende, the brushes with death I described earlier, are viewed in Latin cultures as an event that often precedes miracles. Poet Lorca said they inspire a leap of the imagination toward new life, whether it be in art, culture, or love. Poets will often pray for the *duende* to touch them, so they are able to dive deeply enough into life to bring forth what is most original. It is considered a gift from the muse or the gods, but only if one makes something of it like poetry, music, art, spirituality, love. The brushes with death I experienced within my beloved

195

community catapulted me fully into life. I was more concerned with becoming as present as I could possibly become in every moment of my life than I was with finishing my studies or even graduating. I felt an urgent need to have my arm around what needed to live, to be doing my work fully and immediately, in all moments, not just as a psychotherapist, but in all relationships.

I met with my colleagues to let them know I needed to step forward on the path that took me directly and completely into life, because I had no idea how long life might be for me or anyone else. Though I would not be completing formal analytic training, I felt that I was being well taught by all that life had to bring. I accepted the name that best described what had emerged from my brushes with death: "friend," whose meaning comes from the Middle English *freon, fregon,* or "to love." I would always befriend the life force wherever and whenever I might come across its struggle to come forth, in all its miraculous and ordinary forms in both the plant and animal worlds, through relationship, story, prayer, photographs, poetry; however I might see a way to put my arm around it, I would. And so we closed our time together in a circle with our arms around one another, honoring each one of our struggles and gifts, and the love we would continue to share.

The photographs of trees I had framed and presented to my professional community eventually found homes in local stores and restaurants, stimulating conversations among the customers, many of whom had their own tree stories to add to the collection of nature's stories. After vacationing in Arizona, one of the restaurant owners handed me a photograph of a tree that she had taken when out walking one day. I looked at the image of a trunk that towered over a hundred feet high, but was clearly dead. One of its very powerful lower branches was not only still alive; it had twisted upward into a trunk reaching almost as tall as the original. She had tears in her eyes when she said that finding this tree, reflecting the successful outcome of a life story similar to her own, had set her free of the heartache, finally. After ten years of grieving the loss of her thirty-five-year marriage, she was able to recognize the gift of her own extraordinary life in being able to create another life, just as rich and full, yet very different from the first. She felt gratitude for this miraculous force which had emerged to carry her far beyond her grief into a new and abundant life. Together, we shared the natural gift economy of stories that could never be depleted as long as we passed them along as generously as nature inspired us to do, as long as we perceived the source that connected us in all our diversity, in the many twists and turns of fate.

CHAPTER 20
Like Trees Walking

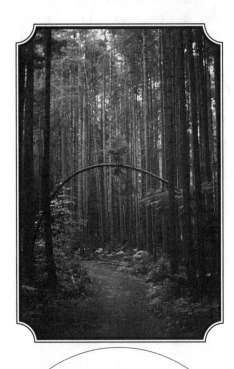

Arch Tree *grows over the trails*
behind South Whidbey High School in Langley, Washington.
At the top of its arch,
a branch has transformed into a tree that now sustains the entire arch
with its topmost branches on the ground.

Chapter 20

After one of our evening meals together, I sat with a group of writing colleagues around the wood-burning stove, where we read aloud to each other from our latest work. I had just finished reading about my walk through Carkeek Park, ending with a description of the hemlock perched atop the old-growth nurse-log with long root legs which made it appear to be walking through the forest. One of the writers surprised all of us by responding to my story with a story from the Bible about how a blind man had been healed by the laying on of hands. She described how the man opened his eyes to see what first looked like trees walking. I felt honored to have this ancient parable join our storyteller's circle, and asked if she would find the passage and read it to us.

From Mark 8:22-26: "They came to Bethsaida, and some people brought to him a blind man whom they begged him to touch. He took the blind man by the hand and led him outside the village. Then putting spittle on his eyes and laying his hands on him, he asked, 'Can you see anything?' The man, who was beginning to see, replied, 'I can see people; they look like trees to me, but they are walking about.' Then he laid his hands on the man's eyes again and he saw clearly; he was cured, and he could see everything plainly and distinctly."

Like Trees Walking, the original title of this book, has been about learning to see differently, which is the gift of my decade-long pilgrimage into nature.

The practice of recognizing healing gifts inherent in nature's stories has been like a walking prayer, a quest to the sacred sites without having to travel thousands of miles to find them. With living altars all around us, we only need to step into our own backyards to touch into the life story of a tree. These gifts grow in city parks, from pots, along the highway, in rugged wilderness, even indoors. They grow everywhere there is a bit of earth and sometimes even from stone. They show us how to see with clear eyes, far beyond our preconceptions about life and healing.

When I first came across the lodge-pole pine that bent and leaned over a trail behind South Whidbey Island High, I was worried about walking under it, even though the trunk arched twenty feet above me. It looked like one of the many tall, flimsy pines in the forest that had accelerated too fast in its race for sunlight, and no longer had the strength to hold its height upright. There were plenty of them folded over in the forest amidst those with sturdier trunks. The one forming a high archway across my path had rested its topmost branches on the ground at the side of the trail, apparently finding stability in a most original way. I wondered how it survived with all its greenery on the ground, and in the shade. A long, productive life did not look possible for this tree.

Yet, when I allowed my eyes to look truly in the way nature had taught me, with beginner eyes, I could see that it was thriving beyond all my expectations. Perhaps it had found enough sunlight from somewhere. I looked along its arching trunk until I noticed, perched at the very top, center point over the trail, what looked to be a Christmas tree growing from it. With the help of sunlight available from the clearing of the trail, a lone branch had transformed into trunk cells so it could turn and grow straight upward into a tree. The arching tree had miraculously given birth to another tree that now stood over six feet tall. Not only was it thriving, but its lush greenery sustained the whole tree. Having found a most creative solution in difficult times, this *fallen* one inspires whoever walks under it.

Later, I heard that the cross-country track team has a great fondness for their "arch tree," as they call it, for encouraging them to see beyond competition. It is a living altar that can be visited time and again as a touchstone for all. I was reminded of the word "genius," which could be traced to its root meaning *genere* (to beget, to bring about new life, originality, a fresh perspective). Nature reveals to us the genius that dwells within the heart of healing, within the life force of every living being, no matter what the life stories might have been in the past. I have learned over my ten-year pilgrimage with nature that the originality of genius can be seen within any moment. Nature has focused my attention more fully on recognizing and appreciating the creative manifestations of life force in the present.

This is quite a dramatic turn of focus, considering that my training and education as a psychotherapist has been directed toward understanding the early bonding patterns and influences in our lives, as if concentrating on the past is the more essential puzzle piece for healing in the present. Clearly, all parts of our lives matter. When I read the story of the arch tree, I don't focus only at its foundation to understand the meaning of its life. I see how it bends at midlife, not only to find and manifest its genius, but to save its life. The gifts of nature have expanded my philosophy of healing far beyond the ancient myth of the wounded healer, and they have opened my spiritual concepts to be all-inclusive, even pantheistic.

Reflecting on all that has happened over the past decade of this pilgrimage into nature, beginning when I stood next to the cedar tree whispering, *Please help me*, there has been a continuous flow, a rhythm of responses from the world of nature. To see and hear them, I had to be fully present, actually immersed in the images and sounds both around me and within. The word "immersion" refers to *being plunged into*, to being completely covered by, as in baptism. As some people feel the sacred blessing of churches, I feel baptized by the life rhythms of the natural world, whether I am absorbed in reading the life story of a tree, listening to the birds, wind, coyotes, or the sound of beach stones turning in the tides.

As I mention in the earlier chapters, I still find myself having in-love feelings, standing in front of the trees that call me to photograph and share their life stories. They are beloved and worth honoring for the generosity of their gifts to humans. But our life stories are intertwined and call for a mutuality that is beneficial to all who live in community. What might we humans offer back to the world of nature to keep this gift economy circulating and generative in the years to come? For the Millennium Celebration, I contributed to this challenge in a small way by writing a haiku poem each day of the year 2000. When read altogether, they reveal the life story of a year in companionship with the natural world. When gathered into shorter clusters, they offer an imagistic walk in the woods for anyone who is not yet able to discover this sacred relationship awaiting them in nature.

In the rain forest,
Green is a wet miracle
of shining mirrors.

Stereophonic
Owls who-whooo from left to right.
Between, we listen.

Night white butterfly
Crosses our path in darkness.
A ribbon of hope.

I trust skunk cabbage.
Yellow fronds emerge from muck.
Show us how to pray.

Like Trees Walking

Coyotes vanish
Before our eyes, blending
Blond tails, branches.

When love is clear-cut,
Stinging nettles find sunlight,
Shelter all new seeds.

Daffodils in snow,
Trumpet sunlight not yet here.
Imagine, they say!

What is trust, but trees
Turning towards hopes of light,
While thriving in shade?

Pantheists, we praise
This moss illuminated
By shimmering light.

From humus, the word
Humiliated brings us
Back to our earth.

Bowing to the ground,
Bowing to the rain, bowing
To the rooting seed.

Index

Index

Index

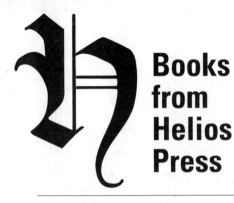

Books from Helios Press

Helios Press and Allworth Press are imprints of Allworth Communications, Inc. Selected titles are listed below.

How to Heal: A Guide for Caregivers
by Jeff Kane, M.D. (paperback, 5 1/2 x 8 1/2, 208 pages, $16.95)

The Inner Source: Exploring Hypnosis, Revised Edition
by Donald S. Connery (paperback, 5 3/8 x 8 1/4, 304 pages, $16.95)

At War with Time: The Wisdom of Western Thought from the Sages to a New Activism for Our Time
by Craig Eisendrath (hardcover, 6 1/4 x 9 1/4, 304 pages, $24.95)

The Dilemma of Psychology: A Psychologist Looks at His Troubled Profession
by Lawrence LeShan, Ph.D. (paperback, 5 1/2 x 8 1/2, 224 pages, $16.95)

The Psychology of War: Comprehending Its Mystique and Its Madness
by Lawrence LeShan, Ph.D. (paperback, 6 x 9, 192 pages, $16.95)

The Medium, the Mystic, and the Physicist: Toward a General Theory of the Paranormal
by Lawrence LeShan, Ph.D. (paperback, 51/2 x 8 1/2, 320 pages, $19.95)

Feng Shui and Money: A Nine-Week Program for Creating Wealth Using Ancient Principles and Techniques
by Eric Shaffert (paperback, 6 x 9, 256 pages, $16.95)

The Secret Life of Money: How Money Can Be Food for the Soul
by Tad Crawford (paperback, 5 1/2 x 8 1/2, 304 pages, $14.95)

What Money Really Means
by Thomas Kostigen (paperback, 6 x 9, 224 pages, $19.95)

The Money Mentor: A Tale of Finding Financial Freedom
by Tad Crawford (paperback, 6 x 9, 272 pages, $14.95)

Please write to request our free catalog. To order by credit card, call 1-800-491-2808 or send a check or money order to Helios Press, 10 East 23rd Street, Suite 510, New York, NY 10010. Include $5 for shipping and handling for the first book ordered and $1 for each additional book. Ten dollars plus $1 for each additional book if ordering from Canada. New York State residents must add sales tax.

To see our complete catalog on the World Wide Web, or to order online, you can find us at
www.heliospress.com.